MAKING
EXCELLENCE
A HABIT

ADVANCE PRAISE FOR THE BOOK

'Dr Mohan's unparalleled contribution to the cause of diabetes is well known, but beneath the innumerable accolades and recognition lies a simple and inspirational story of determination, dedication, resilience, the grit to overcome setbacks and the drive to make a real difference—aspects that resonated with me as a sportsman, and which I am sure will resonate with, enlighten and motivate one and all'—Anil Kumble, former Indian cricketer, coach and commentator

'*Making Excellence a Habit* epitomizes the multifaceted personality of Dr V. Mohan as a doctor, researcher, scientist, teacher, administrator and entrepreneur. The book is highly motivating and inspirational and a must-read for people of all ages as it reveals the ingredients of success based on Dr Mohan's own life. It shows how spirituality and empathy can be seamlessly blended with medicine and science'—V.V.S. Laxman, former Indian cricketer and commentator

'Dr V. Mohan epitomizes excellence in diabetes care. This book is a testimony to his life's dedication to the pursuit of finding answers to the unsolved problems caused by a dreaded disease called diabetes'—Kiran Mazumdar-Shaw, chairperson and managing director of Biocon Limited

'I am very happy to hear that Penguin Random House is publishing the autobiography of Dr V. Mohan, Asia's most iconic diabetologist. Diabetes in India is virtually like an epidemic. Every Indian past the age of fifty is a diabetic unless proven otherwise. Dr Mohan and his passionate team were instrumental in elevating the standards of diabetes care in India. Thank you for creating a monumental document which will be a guiding force for the future generations of medical doctors'—Dr Devi Shetty, cardiac surgeon

MAKING EXCELLENCE A HABIT

The Secret to Building a World-Class Healthcare System in India

DR V. MOHAN

PENGUIN
VIKING

An imprint of Penguin Random House

VIKING

USA | Canada | UK | Ireland | Australia
New Zealand | India | South Africa | China

Viking is part of the Penguin Random House group of companies
whose addresses can be found at global.penguinrandomhouse.com

Published by Penguin Random House India Pvt. Ltd
4th Floor, Capital Tower 1, MG Road,
Gurugram 122 002, Haryana, India

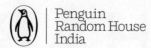

First published in Viking by Penguin Random House India 2021

Copyright © Dr V. Mohan 2021

ISBN 9780670094530

Typeset in Adobe Garamond Pro by Manipal Technologies Limited, Manipal
Printed at Thomson Press India Ltd, New Delhi

www.penguin.co.in

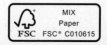

Contents

List of Abbreviations and Acronyms

ADA	American Diabetes Association
CCEBDM	Certificate Course in Evidence-Based Diabetes Mellitus
CUPS	Chennai Urban Population Study
CURES	Chennai Urban Rural Epidemiological Study
DCGI	Drugs Controller General of India
DMDEA	Dr Mohan's Diabetes Education Academy
DMDSC	Dr Mohan's Diabetes Specialities Centre
ENT	Ear, nose and throat
ESRD	End-stage renal disease
ICMR	Indian Council of Medical Research
ICU	Intensive care unit
IDF	International Diabetes Federation
MBBS	Bachelor of Medicine and Bachelor of Surgery
MD	Doctor of Medicine
MDRF	Madras Diabetes Research Foundation
NCDs	Non-communicable diseases
NDEP	National Diabetes Educator Program
NGT	Normal glucose tolerance
NIH	National Institutes of Health
PHFI	Public Health Foundation of India

SSLC	Secondary School Leaving Certificate
TZD	Thiazolidinediones
UAB	University of Alabama at Birmingham
WDF	World Diabetes Foundation

Prologue

It was June 2018. I was in Orlando, Florida, with 15,000 scientists, diabetes and endocrine specialists, nutritionists, educators, nurses and students from all over the globe at the annual meeting of the American Diabetes Association (ADA). The five-day meeting is one of the largest in the world, featuring significant advances in the field of diabetes, and bringing together clinicians and researchers from over 100 countries. I had been attending the meeting since I was a young doctor, one of the many starry-eyed participants watching the proceedings with awe; but not today.

Today was special, a day when the work of the Madras Diabetes Research Foundation and Dr Mohan's Diabetes Specialities Centre at Chennai, India, in helping to raise the standard of care for diabetes for Indians and those in other developing countries, was going to be showcased to the entire medical fraternity. Today was going to be an important milestone, since, for the first time, the ADA, the largest scientific diabetes organization in the world, would be honouring a practising diabetes specialist from India with one of its prestigious international awards. The day was going to be etched in history.

I sat there, experiencing chills and gooseflesh, finding it incredible that I had traversed a journey remarkable enough for a global stage,

when Dr William T. Cefalu, chief scientific officer, ADA, made
the announcement: 'The American Diabetes Association is pleased
to present the 2018 Dr Harold Rifkin Award for Distinguished
International Service in the Cause of Diabetes to Dr Viswanathan
Mohan. Internationally renowned, Dr Mohan has worked tirelessly to
address the challenges of diabetes in India and developing countries.'

After Dr Cefalu's announcement, multiple large screens inside
the auditorium played my pre-recorded acceptance speech video,
in which I explained the work that we at Dr Mohan's centres have
carried out over the years. As the video played across the screens,
I was filled with a sense of humility and gratitude to my father,
Prof. M. Viswanathan, who was the sole reason I took up medicine,
to all my teachers, my family, particularly my late wife, Dr Rema
Mohan, my daughter, Dr Anjana, my son-in-law, Dr Ranjit
Unnikrishnan, my grandson, Pranav, my colleagues at my centre,
numerous collaborators and, most importantly, my spiritual guru
and master, Bhagawan Sri Sathya Sai Baba, without whose guidance
and blessings my life would be incomplete.

Dr Cefalu interrupted my reverie again. 'In recognition of
his outstanding international service in the cause of diabetes,'
he said, 'please welcome our Harold Rifkin Award recipient for
2018, Dr Viswanathan Mohan.' Instantly, the hall came alive with
thunderous applause, especially from the large contingent of Indian
doctors, several of whom were my students. I stood up and walked
confidently to the stage as years of hard work flashed across my
eyes. I received the award from Dr Jane Reusch, the president of
the ADA, and went back to sit close to my family. Soon after the
award ceremony, I was surrounded by colleagues, particularly from
India, as well as several members of the press and media. Multiple
interviews followed.

When I finally got time off, numerous questions started crowding
my head. *Where and when did this journey start? How did I get to where*

I was today? What were the factors that contributed to the success I had achieved in my life? I was overcome with a great desire to know for myself, and to share; to let people know what had worked for me, and what hadn't, so that those with similar dreams, or those who may be embarking on a journey similar to the one that started for me over forty years ago, could find strength and solace in my story.

And as I thought this, my mind travelled to my childhood, to when it all began: with dreams of poetry, not medicine.

1

The Initial Dreams

I have always been delighted at the prospect of a new day, a fresh try, one more start, with perhaps a bit of magic waiting somewhere behind the morning.

—J.B. Priestley, British novelist, playwright and essayist

It was the summer of 1968. I came home after the last day of school, excited that the summer holidays had finally begun. For the next few weeks, I could do whatever I wanted. No, it was not playing cricket or eating the delicious mangoes that India is famous for. I was free to give all my energy and time to my new-found love: English!

Those days we had three streams of schools in Chennai (then known as Madras): the SSLC (Secondary School Leaving Certificate), matriculation and the Anglo-Indian Board of Examinations (now called the Inter-State Board for Anglo-Indian Education). My school deeply valued English, and as the years went by, I grew fascinated with English literature, poetry and essays. We were spellbound when our English teacher taught us the nuances of the language. He would recite with aplomb and poise the poems of Shelley, Wordsworth and Tennyson.

I was enchanted by Percy Bysshe Shelley's description of the moon in his poem, 'The Cloud':

That orbèd maiden with white fire laden,
Whom mortals call the Moon.

William Wordsworth's words after seeing daffodils would resonate whenever I was alone with nature.

I gazed—and gazed—but little thought
What wealth the show to me had brought.

When I read Tennyson's lines in 'The Brook', I could almost hear the sound of bubbling water:

I chatter over stony ways,
*   In little sharps and trebles,*
I bubble into eddying bays,
*   I babble on the pebbles . . .*
I chatter, chatter, as I flow
*   To join the brimming river . . .*

Our English teachers helped us develop a vivid imagination through their classes, and in my spare time, I would try to imitate the writing of the authors and poets I read. And so, during this holiday, I was determined to spend more time with books and immerse myself in literature and poetry. On the last day of school, I returned home with a stack of English classics to read. My father opened the door and, eyeing me with a concerned look, asked me to meet him after dinner so we could 'talk'.

Slowly, laboriously, I went to see my father. He was sitting in his study, wearing his crisp white dhoti and well-starched half-sleeved shirt. He looked impeccably dressed compared to me, a fourteen-year-old boy, standing in a T-shirt and ill-fitting trousers that were a hand-me-down.

With a rather stern visage, he said to me, 'So what is this with your English literature? I see that you're getting very interested. Can't you do it as a pastime?'

With great trepidation I answered, 'No, Dad, this is what I like and this is what I want to do with my life.'

'But is this going to give you a proper job? How are you going to earn your living?'

'I can become a famous writer. I can write books, win awards, travel the world.'

'Remember, Mohan,' he said, with a touch of warmth. 'You might have the talent but not all those who set out to become writers actually succeed. There are other ways in which you can use your writing talent.'

'Like what?'

'Like scientific research. I publish a lot of research papers. If you have a passion for this, you can take up serious writing and spend your life in research.'

I knew my father was egging me on to become a doctor, and I was prepared to protest. 'But I don't think I'll ever make a good doctor. I can't imagine becoming a surgeon and using a knife on someone. I will mess it up.'

My father, too, was prepared with deft responses. 'Who said you have to take up surgery? You can also be a physician.'

Let me backtrack a bit to give you a background of what prompted him to request me to take up medicine as a career.

My father, Professor M. Viswanathan, served as the honorary professor of medicine at the Stanley Medical College and Hospital in Chennai (then known as Madras), the bustling metropolitan city and capital of Tamil Nadu in southern India. In the 1940s, there were no medical colleges in his home state of Kerala, so students who wished to pursue their medical studies had to come to Chennai. In 1940, my father was allotted a seat at the Government Stanley Medical College. He completed his undergraduate and postgraduate medical education in the same college. In 1948, with the support of his teacher and mentor, Dr K.C. Paul, he started the first diabetes clinic in India at Stanley Medical College. That marked the birth of the speciality of diabetology in India and earned him the title of 'Father of Diabetology' in India. This clinic later grew into a department of diabetology and, more recently, was upgraded into a full-fledged Institute of Diabetology. In the late 1960s, changes in government policy meant that my father had to give up his job at Stanley. As he was still relatively young, he shifted his focus on building a private diabetes clinic.

It was this unexpected turn of events that led him to talk to me on that warm summer night in 1968. I was his eldest son and his hopes naturally rested on me to take up medicine and continue his legacy. At that time, starting a private institution devoted to a single speciality, such as diabetes healthcare and research, was unheard of in India. Naturally, I was hesitant.

'But a physician's job is so monotonous,' I argued. 'I've seen you do it, Grandma did it. Just seeing patients the whole day will bore me to death.'

'That's where research comes in,' my father answered. 'You can use your imagination, and who knows, one day you may find a cure for diabetes!' This piqued my interest. 'Remember Frederick Banting and Charles Best were young researchers when they discovered insulin. Why can't you take up some such research on diabetes?'

I had been dreaming about teaching English and writing articles and books. But in that moment, something changed. It didn't help that people of my generation were overwhelmingly obedient to their parents. After a few days of internal battle, I decided to follow my father's wishes. I pacified myself by thinking that I could still fulfil my ambition of becoming a writer, even if I took up medicine. I could write original scientific and review articles besides writing books on medicine and diabetes. In turn, my father promised me that he would help me establish a research centre at the diabetes hospital he was about to establish. A deal was struck that day.

But the shift wasn't easy. Luckily, I spent the whole of the first year of MBBS at the Madras Medical College reading English classics and poetry and writing essays and poems. In a way, my dream of studying English literature was partly fulfilled due to this. This may be one reason why I did not feel too disappointed about giving up the study of English and taking up medicine. From the second year of medicine, I started writing scientific articles and, slowly, started giving it priority. After I got my MBBS degree, I stuck entirely to scientific writing. Indeed, it was this early start in life as a scientific medical researcher that led to the large number of papers that I would eventually publish. Now, when I look back, I have no regrets that I decided to change the course of my life in the summer of 1968.

2

The Winds of Change

When one door closes, another always opens; but we usually look so intently upon the closed door that we do not see the one that has opened.

—Johann Paul Richter, German humorist and prose writer, in the *New England Farmer*, 1909

The anatomy building in the Madras Medical College is popularly referred to as the 'Red Fort'. This red-brick building, built in the Indo-Saracenic style, is enough to induce a sense of awe in every new medical student. When I first saw it in 1971, it reminded me of the building in the movie *Psycho* and frightened me even from the outside.

Every day, when our batch of young medical students entered the building, fresh dead bodies doused in formalin did, too. And my first recollection of entering the anatomy department was the terrible smell of formalin that pervaded the entire place. My close friends, India's future surgeons, relished the anatomy class for the joy of dissecting the various organs in the human body. But I sat away from the corpse, allowing my friends to take charge, while I peeped in occasionally. I was particularly sensitive to the smell of formalin; my nose would twitch, eyes water, and I just couldn't wait to get out of the building.

All these years, I had cultivated the personality of a dreamer, a romantic, and now that I was locked in the stinking Red Fort, I struggled. Anatomy leaves little scope for imagination, and that showed in my exam papers and marks.

I didn't continue the MBBS course without resistance: several times I told my father that I wanted to quit and that this was not what I had planned in life. My father knew my psyche and was patient. He asked me to wait until I started my clinical postings in the third year of MBBS. From then onwards, he assured me, life would be different and I would enjoy studying medicine. I, on my part, intensely disliked anatomy and coped by scribbling poems in the anatomy theatre—poems as dull and depressing as the environment around. I reproduce one below that I wrote in November 1972, during my anatomy posting in second-year MBBS.

Living with the Dead

I have no prejudice against the dead,
*   I rather envy their state*
Our sorrows and troubles scare them not,
*   While our problems they have not.*
Yet every morning as I sit in a hall,
*   Just a foot away from a corpse,*
And occasionally cut his unfortunate veins,
*   I feel a pang of detest and sorrow.*

I feel that had he been at all alive,
*   He would have staunchly protested;*

Not even for science, to save humanity
     Would he have agreed to cut up his body.
This feeling haunts me time and again,
     As I sit close to him and use my knife;
So instead of chopping up dead men,
     I'd prefer to deal with a man alive.

Meanwhile, I also escaped anatomy by turning my attention to physiology and biochemistry—particularly reading and rereading the famous physiology book by Best and Taylor. As a young medical student at the University of Toronto, Charles Best had worked as an assistant to the surgeon Dr Frederick Banting and contributed to the discovery of insulin, which had led to the Nobel Prize for Medicine in 1923.

From the second year of MBBS onwards, I had, due to my new-found interest in diabetes, already started reading quite a bit about the disease and was passionate about Banting and Best's work. Around the same time, I heard about what was called the 'Prize Exam'. Apart from the university exams, Madras Medical College conducted these prize exams for academically sharper students. It was in 1972 that the semester system was introduced for the first time for the MBBS course in Tamil Nadu. At the end of the first semester of second-year MBBS, we appeared for a university exam that covered half the portion of each subject, i.e. anatomy, physiology and biochemistry. But for those who wished to appear for the prize exam, which was held at the very end of second-year MBBS, the portions of both semesters had to be studied. As it was bad enough studying for one semester, only a few students opted to appear for this exam.

Out of a class of hundred, five signed up for the anatomy prize exam; but for the physiology prize exam, it was just me. Every day, for those one and a half years, I earnestly prepared for the physiology prize. At first, I went to the department library to look up the portions and previous years' question papers. A mix of thirty-five to forty questions were repeated year after year and so it struck me that if I prepared for these, I would walk away with the prize. I bought several books on physiology—almost everything I could lay my hands on, and borrowed some, too. In all, I had seventeen books on physiology, and from these I created copious notes for all those forty questions, where sometimes each answer ran to several pages—a mini thesis of sorts.

At home, my father noticed how much time I was devoting to the prize-exam preparation and was worried that I was neglecting the other subjects. One day he took me aside and told me, 'Mohan, I am putting down a condition; you can only study for the physiology prize after you finish studying your regular portions for the university exam.'

Thus began my sleepless nights. Every evening, I would study for the university exams from 6 p.m. to midnight, and after midnight, I would pick up my physiology books. At 3 a.m., I would retire to sleep for three hours and would get up at 6 a.m. to leave for college. I maintained this oppressive schedule for over a year. An associate professor in the physiology department noticed this madness. He told me, 'Mohan, these prize exams are not worth putting in so much effort for. Don't burn yourself out. Take it easy.'

But I had always been competitive, eager to prove my mettle; and by this time, I was almost in a state of delirium. Succeeding in the prize exam seemed like the most important thing in my life.

A day before the exam, the professor of physiology announced in the class that they had only received one name for the physiology prize; he forced the five anatomy-prize students to appear for the physiology exam and warned them to 'be prepared to fail in physiology in the university exams' in case they didn't. The students were reluctant but eventually agreed due to the professor's threat. Here I was, with a whole year's preparation behind me, and answers to all possible questions, and my five friends who hadn't even looked at the syllabus. After the exam began, four of them left within a few minutes while I forced a friend to remain for half an hour. There was no time limit for the prize exam and I filled answer sheets for the next five and a half hours. I was thrilled that all the questions that were asked were the ones I had prepared elaborate answers for. Eventually, the invigilator forced me to stop writing. He shook my hand and told me that I had written enough—almost a thesis of over a hundred pages. 'The prize is yours, it's yours,' he said, and congratulated me.

But when the results were announced, the award went to someone else. I had written elaborate answers to every question, some of which my friends had not even attempted, and yet, I was denied the award. Even in the only subject I liked, I had tasted failure, and this came as a major blow to me. That day, I went home and told my father that enough was enough, that I couldn't stomach it any more and was quitting medicine.

My father sat me down and spoke to me for an hour. 'I never appeared for these prize exams and yet I made a success of myself,' he said. 'I told you not to waste your time on what doesn't matter. Now, I will give you a plan which, if you follow, will ensure that you won't go wrong, I assure you.' Despite the sting of failure, I was prepared to listen. 'Forget about the prize exams or the quest for medals. Focus on research. You seem to have a bent of mind for research and writing. Medical students don't do research and hence you will have no competition. Very soon, you will carve out a niche for yourself that no one else would have.'

I heard him at that moment and thought deeply for days. Perhaps, I thought, he was right, and once again, I decided to obey him. I began to focus on research and writing scientific papers. I made a choice, and abstract poetry left me; scientific research slowly became a passion, which, to this day, it continues to be.

But my zeal wasn't just self-induced; it was demonstrative of the undeniable role one's peers or environment play in shaping one's life. My zeal was propelled by the kind of environment I enjoyed at the Madras Medical College. In my class, some of the brightest minds studied together, and as the students started interacting, we knew that we were an exceptional batch. The competition was so fierce that no one student could walk away with all the prizes and medals. We didn't just study, we also participated in several extracurricular activities from athletics and sports to fine arts and dramatics. And at the end of the course, we didn't just grow into responsible, mature adults, we also fell in love and found life partners within the class— about eight couples, or 16 per cent of the class, married each other! This wasn't the only record. Many more records were broken by my batchmates.

For instance, the college awarded the Bannerman Medal to a student who was able to score at least 70 per cent in the microbiology-prize exam. If there was no one who scored as much, the prize was awarded but not the medal. It was a rare feat to receive the medal, and in several of the earlier batches, no student had been awarded it. In my batch, five students scored 70 per cent and the college had to introduce several rounds of tiebreakers to decide the eventual recipient of the Bannerman Medal.

At the college's 175th year, they decided to honour the best batch in the college's long history. Several batches, including our immediate juniors and seniors, applied, but we were unanimously chosen as the best batch. It wasn't particularly surprising because our batch had set records that none of the others could match. Three of my classmates went on to be awarded the Padma Shri, the fourth-highest civilian award awarded by the Government of India; three received the Dr B.C. Roy Award, the highest honour bestowed on a medical doctor by the Medical Council of India; several became presidents of national medical associations in their own specialties;

and some even became presidents of the Asian associations of their speciality. One became the vice chancellor of the prestigious Tamil Nadu Dr M.G.R. Medical University in Tamil Nadu, and several eventually became professors and teachers. In addition, the number of research papers collectively published by the class was a record, and we were able to boast of several other honours and laurels. The most important lesson this taught me was that peer pressure or, simply, the company one keeps, definitely helps one succeed. And it was certainly the excellence I saw all around that pushed me to aspire for the pinnacle of success in medicine and research.

3

The New Passion

Nothing in the universe can stop you from letting go and starting over.

—Guy Finley, bestselling self-help writer and spiritual teacher

A number of people in my family are doctors. My paternal grandmother, Dr M. Madhavi Amma, was a general practitioner in Irinjalakuda, a small town near Trichur (now Thrissur) in Kerala. I would spend my summer holidays at her house watching the long queue of patients waiting to see her. My grandmother, a strict disciplinarian but an equally kind-hearted person, was one of the very few women of her generation to practise medicine. Years later, after she retired from practice, she came to live with us in Chennai for a few years. Towards the end of her life, she expressed a desire to return to her hometown. Initially, this was met with a lot of resistance from the family, as they felt that she would have access to better medical care in Chennai. However, she kept pleading with all of us to let her return to her place of birth. One day, when I was alone with her, I asked her why she was so keen to return to Irinjalakuda. Her eyes lit up as she felt the first ray of hope.

'Mohan,' she told me in a soft voice, 'in Chennai, I will die like a stranger. In Irinjalakuda, I will die a queen.'

That settled the issue. I told all the family members that I would shoulder the responsibility of taking her to Kerala.

When we arrived, the whole town turned up to pay their respects to the first doctor in their community. It was an incredible sight, people queuing up just to get a glimpse of her or a word with her. She spent the entire day smiling and speaking to her old friends and acquaintances. The following day she passed away peacefully. Just as she had predicted, hundreds of people attended the funeral. I was happy that my grandma's last wish had been fulfilled.

My paternal aunt, Dr Subhadra Nair, is a renowned obstetrician and gynaecologist, who, now, at the time of writing this book, is in her eighties and still active in her practice. One of my uncles is a well-known cardiologist. As I have noted earlier, my father was perhaps the first diabetologist in India. Both my daughter and son-in-law are diabetologists. This means we have four generations of doctors in the family and three generations of diabetologists! My friends often joke that while we know that diabetes is common in some families, it appears that diabetology also tends to appear in other families. But when people tell me that diabetes runs in their family, I, too, joke with them: it's because no one runs in your family.

After my father convinced me to take up medicine, I started focusing not just on medicine but also on diabetes. The first step in the long journey was to opt for science in my pre-university course which, at that time, was a prerequisite for applying to a medical college. I joined Loyola College and, as compared to my father, lived a comfortable life. But how my father raised us taught me what is easily forgotten: the value of money.

My paternal grandfather died when my father was nine years old, and throughout his student years, my father lived frugally, being able to afford luxuries like ice cream only once or twice during the five-year course. As he was brought up in such trying circumstances, he was a strict disciplinarian and acutely careful with money. When we were children, he would ensure that we were given the exact change needed for our day-to-day living.

I studied at St Mary's High School in George Town in Chennai, and the bus fare for a trip to Royapuram, where I lived at that time, was 50 paisa (half a rupee or less than 1 cent). When I requested money to buy storybooks, my father was reluctant, fearing I could be distracted from my studies. I would therefore walk home every day to save the bus fare. At the end of the week, I would have saved enough money to buy a storybook, which I would finish reading during the weekend, and then start the process all over again the following week.

Like my father, I continued to be frugal well after school. From my second year of medical college, I started working part-time with my father in his clinic. I would spend time learning to do research and analysing data, creating slides for his lectures and helping him write research papers and chapters in various textbooks All this of course gave me a head start in my future field of specialization. By the time I had completed my undergraduate medical education, I had already written twenty research papers. As our economic standing improved, I also started travelling with my father—initially, around the country and, soon, all around the world. This exposed me to the work done on diabetes at various research centres and universities, nationally and internationally. Needless to say, my self-confidence got a huge boost.

But my passion for college and research work was not limited to diabetes. My initial years in medical college are special to me for another reason as well: it was then that I met my wife, Rema.

One day, in the first week of our medical course, I was travelling to college on a local bus. It was a pleasant August day and the air had been freshened by soft drizzles of rain. Autumn has always fascinated me; I had seen movies like *Dr Zhivago* which show the changing colours of the leaves in autumn—green, yellow, orange, gold and red. It was the ideal time of the year for romance.

I was sitting by the window, casually looking around, when I noticed an extremely beautiful girl sitting a couple of seats away from me. I was instantly smitten. I had heard of 'love at first sight' but had only witnessed it in movies. My classmates saw me looking at her and the teasing began. I was preoccupied—trying to guess where she lived and where she might be disembarking. A few minutes later, my college bus-stop arrived, and my heart skipped a beat when I saw her rise to alight from the bus. My friends winked at me, while I ignored them and quickly got off the bus too. I crossed the road to go to the college and oh, wonder of wonders, she also crossed the road. Only then did it strike me that she was my college mate.

I later found out that her name was Rema. She studied in a different section of the class, which explained why I had not seen her earlier. Thus began a long period of my attempt at courtship, which went on for five years. I tried several techniques to talk to her, including offering her my carefully prepared notes on various subjects. She was always polite but extremely difficult to read. This is reflected in one of the poems I wrote at the time, titled 'Unrequited Love', from which I reproduce a stanza:

> Days fled past like frightened cattle,
>   With Love, did her admirer battle;
> Weeks turned to months without a word
>   His obsession pierced him like a sword.

I was in love and was eager to find out everything I could about her; it turned out that she was distantly related to me. I began to attend family functions like weddings where I was sure she would also be present. Rema's father worked at the United States Information

Services at the time; this gave me an opportunity to contact him on the pretext of borrowing books from the American Library. Much later, Rema confessed that her father was impressed with that 'studious boy in your class who spent so much time reading' from pretty much the beginning.

In classrooms, I found myself unable to pay attention until I had seen Rema enter adorned in a beautiful sari (she was always impeccably dressed) and a large *bottu* (bindi) on her forehead. This inspired me to write several poems about her; a couple of stanzas from one such piece are reproduced below:

> The pulsating heart quickened its beat
>> Could the heart feel what the mind controlled?
> Every channel in the complex brain vibrated
>> With the spasm, the uncontrollable emotion.
>
> And then the chance meeting;
>> Days of eager anticipation and fervent prayer
> Raised hopes of fluttering hearts and joyous union.

When we were doing our house surgeoncy (compulsory internship) after clearing our final MBBS exams, I decided I had to know whether Rema had the same feelings for me or not. One day, I approached her and told her which medical unit I had been posted to for my internship and requested her to apply to the same unit. I told myself that if she accepted my request, she was interested in me; if not, my attempts were futile.

A week passed and the medical posting was drawing near. On the first day, I was waiting with bated breath, remembering all the gods I could, when she turned up. 'I insisted that I should be posted in this unit,' she said, her eyes sparkling, 'How can I say no to you?' The rest, as they say, is history. I proposed to her at the end of the house surgeoncy and soon we were engaged. On 7 February 1979, Rema and I were married. I was blessed to be with the love of my life, for the rest of our lives.

Years later Rema told me, 'Mohan, I always had deep feelings for you. But I was scared to take the big step. That time when you asked me to marry you during the house-surgeoncy posting was the turning point. And I will never regret that decision as long as I live.'

Two years later, we completed our post-graduation in internal medicine (me) and ophthalmology (her), after which we both joined my father as full-time consultants. Between 1981 and 1991, we devoted ourselves to building the M.V. Hospital for Diabetes and Diabetes Research Centre in Royapuram, which was the earliest institution devoted to diabetes healthcare and research in India. The work was difficult because doing research in a private institution with no funding was a great challenge. However, recognition soon came from various quarters. The Government of India recognized our centre as a research foundation, thus enabling income-tax exemptions. We directed most of our clinical earnings to research and, slowly but steadily, built the research facilities. While I was conducting clinical studies on diabetes, Rema decided to devote her life to the study of diabetic eye diseases (diabetic retinopathy), and was one of the earliest doctors in India to do so.

In 1984, Rema and I got an opportunity to work with the world-renowned expert in diabetic retinopathy, Dr Eva Kohner, at the Hammersmith Hospital and Royal Postgraduate Medical School in London. Rema had obtained a small grant from the British Society for the Prevention of Blindness, which barely covered our house rental. We did struggle a lot financially as I shall explain below. However, this was an extremely productive period of our lives as we were able to take our research to the next level. I also worked with Professor Hugh Mather at the Ealing Hospital in Southall, studying the differences in the clinical profiles of diabetes in South Asians and Europeans.

For years we had known that South Asians had an increased susceptibility to type 2 diabetes. But the reason for this had remained an enigma. My studies in the UK showed, for the first time, that Indians have increased insulin resistance compared to matched groups of white Europeans. This was one of the several unique features of the so-called 'South Asian' or 'Asian Indian Phenotype' which would come to be described over the years by research emerging from India. My colleague Dr Patrick Sharp and I conducted euglycemic clamp studies (a test by which we keep the glucose levels constant and see how insulin is used up to achieve this) and proved that Indians had higher insulin resistance. While at Hammersmith Hospital, I also worked in the biochemistry laboratory, running insulin and C-peptide tests on my own, which provided an excellent opportunity to learn about the quality control of various laboratory procedures. Thus, the one year I spent in the UK was remarkably productive, seeing the publication of over a dozen papers in peer-reviewed journals and my first brush with highly rated international journals. Rema also published some excellent papers with Dr Eva Kohner on diabetic retinopathy during this time.

However, if you think that our life in London was a bed of roses, think again. During the first few months, we struggled due to lack of money. In those days, foreign exchange was in short supply in India, and all we received for our year's stay in the UK was about 500 US dollars. I managed to get a little money from an Indian foundation but soon that also ran out. Our first winter outside India was harsh. Rema, Anjana (Anju), our three-year-old daughter, and I were all huddled up in one room as we could only afford the heating for that room. I was able to borrow a little money from a friend but that was also fast running out.

We told our boss, Dr Eva Kohner, about our condition and she said I was welcome to apply anywhere for additional funding. With little hope of even getting a reply, I wrote to the Wellcome Trust explaining my position. I was pleasantly surprised to receive a letter from Dr Bridget Ogilvie, vice president of the Wellcome Trust, asking me to meet her. At our meeting, she asked me only one question: 'Mohan, how do we know that you will return to India and not stay on permanently in the UK?' When she heard about my plans of setting up a research centre for diabetes in India, her eyes widened in admiration. She immediately sanctioned a Wellcome Trust Fellowship, something that even those who lived in the UK would struggle to get these days. This marked the end of our financial troubles. We enjoyed the rest of our stay in the UK—apart from the period being academically highly productive, we also spent time driving all around the country in our cheap third-hand car.

Around the time we were getting ready to leave the UK, around the middle of 1985, came the good news that I had been awarded the prestigious Alexander von Humboldt Foundation Fellowship in Germany. This gave us an opportunity to spend a year at the University of Ulm, working with the world-renowned diabetes expert Prof. E.F. Pfeiffer and his wife, Dr Margaret Pfeiffer, who, luckily for Rema, was a specialist in diabetic eye disorders. After completing our two-year stint abroad, we returned to work at my father's centre in Royapuram. However, things had changed while we were abroad. During the subsequent four years that we spent in Royapuram with my father, Rema and I felt strongly that it was time to enter uncharted waters—to start our own journey in diabetes healthcare and research.

4

The Magic of Serendipity

The universe is always speaking to us . . . sending us little messages, causing coincidences and serendipities, reminding us to stop, to look around, to believe in something else, something more.

—Nancy Thayer, American novelist

In August 1991, Rema and I left my father's centre to start our own. However, we were under huge financial pressure. During our time with my father, we used to donate most of our earnings to research. So when we left the comforts of a salaried job, we did not have enough money. You could say that we had walked out just with our stethoscopes! Rema and I together had about Rs 80,000 in the bank. But the problem was much deeper. Rema had taken a huge bank loan to set up the eye department at my father's centre, which had thrown us into heavy debt.

As the pressure to repay the bank mounted, we realized that we had hit rock bottom. We tried to pacify ourselves thinking that once you reach this low depth, you cannot go any lower, so you have nowhere to go but up. And luckily, several of our friends and patients trusted us and supported us with the funds and resources needed to set up our new clinic. Most of all, I had Rema's support and willpower.

'Mohan, these are passing clouds,' she would say. 'A bright future awaits us. You mark my words.'

On 1 September 1991, we started a diabetes clinic on the ground and first floors of a four-storeyed building on Royapettah High Road in south Chennai. The owner had promised us that he would rent us the two additional floors in a year's time. For reasons best known to him, he broke his promise and refused to give us the upper two floors when they fell vacant. With the number of patients steadily increasing, we were rapidly running out of space. We hired two floors of a nearby hospital to admit our inpatients. But it was inconvenient to run the practice in two locations with separate outpatient and inpatient services. At that point, we decided to take the plunge and look for land to build our own hospital with both services under one roof.

Time and again, life throws challenges at you when you cannot see what lies ahead. That's when you must hold on to your dreams and not give up. Setting up Dr Mohan's Diabetes Specialities Centre (DMDSC) was our dream, and one that we didn't want to give up at any cost, regardless of the hurdles. And in order to achieve that, we had to first raise funds to purchase the land. Again, we had no one to turn to, except our patients and friends who were willing to invest in our dream. While we were scrambling to raise funds, we realized that we didn't have any money ourselves and therefore wouldn't have ownership in our own hospital. We were struggling, trying to find a way to get the money needed to buy the land (and then the building), and as time went by, we almost gave up hopes of setting up our own hospital.

A couple of weeks passed and, one day, a patient who happened to be the chairman of a big financial company came to see me for treatment. After the consultation, I showed him the brochure of the proposed hospital building, hoping to interest him in investing a small sum of money. To my surprise, he took a look at the brochure and said, 'How much money do you need, doctor? I am prepared to give you the whole amount.' I was taken aback and said I would get back to him. I went home and discussed the offer with Rema. As this person was a total stranger, we were hesitant about borrowing a large sum of money from him. However, if we decided to trust him and take the money, we could buy the land straightaway. Rema and I discussed the pros and cons and decided to take a leap of faith.

Rema said, 'Go for it, Mohan. What's the worst that can happen? He may say no. Nothing is lost. Let's take our chance!'

The next day, I went to see this gentleman in his office. I asked him if he would be willing to give us the money as a personal loan; he readily agreed to this and wrote out cheques for the entire amount. I promised him we would repay him with interest but that it might take a long time to return the principal amount. He simply said, 'Take your time, doctor.'

Looking back at this incident, I have to thank that gentleman (almost a complete stranger at the time) from the bottom of my heart, for without those cheques that he so graciously wrote us, we would never have been able to purchase the land and build the hospital or any of the other institutions we have today.

Thus began the journey of DMDSC in Gopalapuram in the heart of Chennai, which continues to be our headquarters even today. We soon started expanding and, now, at the time of writing this book, we have fifty-two branches of DMDSC spread across thirty-five cities and nine states of India, and are still growing.

Alongside the growth of DMDSC, our other institutions were also making rapid progress. The Madras Diabetes Research Foundation (MDRF), the research wing of the organization, was growing equally rapidly and making inroads into new areas of research. The education wing, Dr Mohan's Diabetes Education

Academy (DMDEA), meanwhile, started various courses related to the speciality of diabetology. These supporting sister institutions were in fact the reason we were able to expand our clinical services in the first place. They also added greatly to our growing stature in the field of diabetology, both nationally and internationally.

One never knows how a meeting with a stranger can turn one's life around. A fortuitous interaction with someone can open up new possibilities in life which we might have never even considered. And what appears to happen by chance can have a profound and beneficial influence on one's life. What matters is whether you believe that that opportunity will do its magic. Most people would let their doubts get the better of them. Learning from this experience, I would say, why not take a chance? Some people call it kismet, or destiny. Some refer to it as 'serendipity', which means 'the occurrence and development of events by chance in a happy or beneficial way'. I am a great believer in serendipity, which, I believe, is not merely restricted to the most difficult time of your life. In fact, the real magic of serendipity can be experienced and appreciated when you are already happy and least expect more goodness to follow, like what happened to me in 1998.

Rema and I were in Barcelona, Spain, to attend the annual meeting of the European Association for the Study of Diabetes. During one of the coffee breaks, I met an American doctor. He asked me where I was from and introduced himself as Prof. Michael (Mike) Steffes, a well-known physician and researcher from the University of Minnesota at Minneapolis. He had done pioneering work in pancreas transplantation reversing diabetic kidney and eye complications. When he heard I hailed from India, he asked me whether I knew Prof. Gundu Rao, a close friend of his. To be honest, at the time, I had not heard of the man. Gundu, as he is popularly known, was originally from Karnataka but was then working at the University of Minnesota. When Mike told me that he was coming to India a few weeks later to attend a meeting Gundu was organizing in New Delhi, we immediately exchanged business cards.

After returning to Minneapolis, Mike promptly introduced me to Gundu, who had been championing the cause of atherosclerosis and had published several research papers and books on the subject. Gundu invited me to give a talk at the meeting of the South Asian Society on Atherosclerosis and Thrombosis in Delhi. I accepted his invitation as I could use the opportunity to catch up with Mike. After delivering my talk, I had more than an hour to spare before my flight and so decided to attend a lecture on cardiology in the adjoining room. But the speaker was extremely unimpressive. I lost interest and looked around the room. Sitting next to me was a young doctor from the US, who looked equally bored. I whispered to him, 'This is really boring, isn't it? Shall we step outside for a cup of coffee?' He immediately agreed, relieved to find an excuse to get out of the room. As we sat sipping our coffees, we introduced ourselves. He was Dr Jerome Markowitz, a young cardiologist from the University of Alabama at Birmingham (UAB), and this was his first trip to India. I told him about our diabetes centre and my research interests. Jerome became very interested and mentioned that he had a spare day and wondered whether he could make a trip to Chennai. Soon, Jerome was at our centre and gave a brilliant talk on preventive cardiology and the effect of depression on the heart.

After discussions with our group, Jerome offered to help set up some research investigations which he was doing at UAB. He also proposed that he and I write a research grant together. After a couple of visits to each other's centres, we submitted a grant proposal to the Fogarty International Centre division of the National Institutes of Health (NIH) in the US. The grant was to set up a teaching course at our centre in Chennai on the prevention and control of non-communicable diseases (NCDs) like diabetes and coronary heart disease. Within a few months, we received the good news that the grant had been approved. Unfortunately, along with that, came some really terrible news. Jerome had been diagnosed with pancreatic cancer, and the prognosis did not look good. During an earlier visit to his centre in Alabama, Jerome had introduced me to Prof. Dale Williams, professor of biostatistics and preventive medicine at UAB. Jerome quickly transferred the grant to Dale, who agreed to be the principal investigator from the US side, in place of Jerome. Within a few months, sadly, Jerome passed away.

But the work went on. Dale and Prof. Cora (Beth) Lewis from UAB and Prof. Myron Gross from Minneapolis (and a colleague of Mike Steffes and Gundu Rao) jointly conducted this training course at our centre. When joint research and training grants are funded between the US and India, the usual format is that the grant pays for a couple of scholars from India to go to the US to complete their PhD. It turns out that most of them, after completing their degree, continue their postdoctoral work in the US and rarely come back to India—a classic example of the 'brain drain' phenomenon. We decided to reverse this trend by developing a unique model whereby the US faculty came to teach in India, and in this manner, we reached out to many more institutions domestically—medical colleges, research centres, universities and health departments.

When our Indian scientists or students did go to the US as part of the grant, it was only for a short-term training period of four to eight weeks. We were thus enabling a 'reverse brain-drain' situation which would help us in capacity building within the country. The grant ran successfully for its first term of five years and was then renewed for an additional five years, and then another five. Within an overall span of five years, over 5250 community medicine and public health specialists, faculty, postgraduate and undergraduate students from ninety-six medical colleges, from almost all the Indian states, were trained in the prevention and control of NCDs.

The MDRF–UAB training programme turned out to become the largest training course in the prevention of NCDs ever conducted in India!

If we now look back on the series of events as they unfolded, it is humbling to note that it all started with a casual meeting between Mike Steffes and myself at a conference in Barcelona. This is the magic and power of serendipity!

When people meet, apparently casually, they have no way of knowing what the future holds. Are these incidents random? Is it fate caused by the position of our astrological stars, as some people believe? Are these mere coincidences, or part of a divine plan? No matter what your belief is, make use of the magic of serendipity, of chance, as it might be the start of a new chapter or indeed even a new life for you. Grab every opportunity you have. You may not get it again.

5

Focus and You Will Achieve

My success, part of it, certainly, is that I have focused in on a few things.

—Bill Gates, American business magnate, software developer, investor and philanthropist

The power of focus was first taught to me in school. One of my teachers conducted an experiment that left a lasting impression on me. He took us out into the sun and held out a piece of paper in his hand. We stood there for some time in the hot, humid and sultry Chennai heat. Soon, all of us started sweating, but nothing happened to the paper that our teacher held in his hand. With the dexterity of a magician, he took out a magnifying glass from his pocket. He then focused the rays of the sun through the magnifying glass until it became a small yellow and, later, a red spot on the paper. Within a few minutes, it started burning and soon the entire paper was ashes. After the show was over, he triumphantly declared to us, 'Look at the power of focusing on something. The sun was there. The sun's rays were there. The paper was there. And yet nothing happened. But when we focused the sun's rays on to a point, its power was magnified several hundredfold and so the heat of the sun became powerful enough to burn the paper.'

Our mind, like the sun, is very powerful. Our thoughts can make or break us. Most often, however, our thoughts are uncontrolled, our mind unfocused, and hence we fail to harness the power within the mind, particularly the subconscious mind. But through practice we can begin to focus our mind on an object or on something that we wish to achieve. It could be academics, our future, a job, a holiday, anything for that matter. The moment we start focusing our mind on something, its power increases infinitely. Suddenly, we are able to do things we never thought we could. We are able to achieve what seemingly look like superhuman things.

There is no use if you have all the energy in the world but you spread yourself too thin. You need to act like a magnifying glass which collects energy from the sunlight and focuses it on a single point. The Large Hadron Collider, it is said, uses 10,000 superconducting magnets to keep the protons guided and focused. Wow! That's 'focus' with a capital F.

My early introduction to the speciality of diabetology, thanks to my father, helped me focus on what I wanted to do quite early in life. Right from my second year of medical college, I would repeatedly ask myself, 'How is this going to help me as a diabetologist?' For example, when we had to study anatomy, physiology and biochemistry, I focused more on physiology and biochemistry, reading much more than an average medical student would. This went on throughout my medical course and helped me develop a passion for subjects like pharmacology, therapeutics, medicine and nutrition. I would read entire textbooks related to my future field of specialization, firmly believing that this would stand me in good stead in the future. And, looking back, I must admit that it did. It put me far ahead of the others. Added to this was the fact that I started writing and publishing research articles on diabetes.

I also made it a point to read the latest issues of scientific journals. It was with this very narrow focus that I went through my entire undergraduate and postgraduate medical studies. Since then it has been my conviction that people who had focus did better in their careers and life in general.

My father always insisted that I focus on the task at hand, and it was this habit of honing my focus that helped me learn many skills from him. I started applying these clinical skills early in my career even as an undergraduate medical student and supplemented this with extensive reading of the literature available on diabetes. My father used to treat the records of his patients with the utmost reverence and would ask me to pay attention to them as well. To establish this quality in me, I made patients' case notes my Bhagavad Gita, Quran and Bible. By poring through the case notes, clinical records and investigations of thousands of patients, I acquired deep knowledge about diabetes. These numbers, initially a few hundred, ran into the thousands and then hundreds of thousands. In the initial years, medical records were manually managed, which meant that one's clinical aptitude was honed in the process.

I would also spend time in the laboratory conducting my own experiments. This meant that I was acquiring a combination of both clinical and laboratory skills. Unwavering focus was at the centre of this and, soon enough, I could, with reasonable accuracy, diagnose what type of diabetes a patient walking into my office had. For example, if a very thin, undernourished patient walked in, one could almost be sure that he had a secondary form of diabetes called fibrocalculous pancreatic diabetes, in which stones would be found in the pancreas. My students and fellows would be astonished when I would tell them that a particular patient could have pancreatic stones, and an hour later the X-ray would confirm it.

My knowledge was tested in 2019, when I was asked to take a class for the MD postgraduate students at a medical college.

A bunch of eager young graduates in general medicine discussed the case study of a middle-aged woman with diabetes and chronic liver disease. We discussed at length all the clinical signs and symptoms of the woman and, finally, I asked for the patient's case notes. The students had not brought the case notes or the results of the various laboratory tests with them. But before a student ran to fetch them, I wanted to check my own clinical skills. So I predicted the various clinical and biochemical investigations such as the liver function tests, haemoglobin level and ultrasound findings to the remaining students. A few minutes later, when the results arrived, all of them were astounded to see how close my predictions were to reality. Yes, admittedly, this is not possible in every case and there is certainly a possibility of human error. And that is why I always teach my students that 'two plus two' is very rarely four in biology or medicine. It can be 3.5 or 4.5 because of human variation. But as a clinician and researcher, and after having gone through hundreds of thousands of case records, one can fairly confidently predict the clinical and biochemical findings and outcomes in various situations.

However, focus does not mean that you can do only one thing well in your life. Some of the greatest geniuses to have graced the earth were known to be extremely multitalented. Leonardo da Vinci, Michelangelo, Newton and Goethe were all men of multiple talents but still had intense focus and enjoyed sustained productivity. In modern times, Elon Musk can be said to be a great example of a person who has been able to achieve success in multiple areas.

However, there is no denying the fact that focus is a very important prerequisite to achieving anything in life. Setting specific goals from time to time helps us plan our life and give it a purpose. Often, though, life twists and turns, distracting us from our goals, and we temporarily lose the momentum that we had so carefully built up. Trying to stay focused on the goal on such occasions is often a bigger challenge than attaining that goal itself.

But when you find your rhythm and start thinking seriously about something, what you are doing, in reality, is that you are focusing your mind on achieving that goal. The moment you start doing that, you will find new opportunities coming your way. You will find closed doors magically and miraculously opening. With every passing day, week, month and year, you will move closer and closer to your goal. One way in which you can train your mind to focus is through meditation. When you meditate, you are focusing your mind on a single point. This not only calms the mind and gives you total peace but also sharpens your intellect and helps you dream. In your dreams, you build an image of what you really want in life. The more and more you begin to focus on that, as if by magic, the very thing you desire starts appearing, and if you continue to focus on it, very soon, what you dreamt of becomes a reality.

There is no prescribed age to start this exercise. Obviously, the younger you are when you start training your mind to focus, the more you will achieve in life. However, at any stage of your life, you can ask yourself: *What is it that you want to achieve over the next five, ten or more years?* As you begin to think about this, ideas will come to you. You then start focusing on those ideas and bingo! You have achieved your goal!

6

The Road to Resilience

*Don't judge me by my success, judge me by how many times I fell
down and got back up again.*

—Nelson Mandela, South African anti-apartheid
revolutionary, political leader and philanthropist

In 1971, I joined Loyola College in Chennai for my pre-university
course, which is a prerequisite to entering a medical college. Loyola
is consistently ranked among the top institutions in India. In my
class at Loyola, in the science section alone, there were several other
toppers from different school boards who were converging in the
same pre-university course. The competition therefore was intense.
Back then, this course decided your career. If you were aspiring to
become a doctor, it was imperative to pass your pre-university exams
with flying colours, or you simply had to give up on your dream.

As luck would have it, during that critical year at Loyola, I
developed several illnesses. First, I developed infective hepatitis
(jaundice), which took away a whole month. I came back to college
for two days, after which I fell sick once again. This time, it was
chickenpox (varicella) and I was confined in bed for another two

weeks. Following that I was down with malaria, which meant another two weeks of classes gone. Overall, of the entire eight- or nine-month duration of the course, I was at home, in bed, for nearly two months of it! By the time I recovered from all these illnesses, barely two months remained for the final examination. I was mentally and physically weak and exhausted. At this point, I nearly gave up. There was no way, I thought, I would be able to take the exams, let alone compete with the state rank-holders in the class.

When I finally came back, Prof. V.A. Murthy, who was our zoology professor and an erudite scholar and scientist, asked me to meet him after class. He asked me, with great concern, where I had disappeared all these days. I clearly remember the look in his eyes, which were filled with love and compassion but also concern. I told him, 'Sir, my career is over. I have been down with various illnesses and have missed two months of classes. I have no hope of even writing the exam. I feel like giving up.' To my surprise, he said, 'No, Mohan, don't give up. Are you ready to sacrifice your lunch for the next one month? If you are ready to do this, I will personally coach you and help you make up for all the classes you missed.' I immediately agreed, grateful for his offer.

For the next one month, Professor Murthy intensively coached me in zoology and even enlisted another professor to teach me botany. These were the two most important subjects, requiring very high marks to get a medical seat. As a result of this personal coaching, I improved rapidly. Within a few weeks, I could see that I was catching up with my peers.

By the next internal examination, I was on par with the toppers in the class. And finally came the university examination. I knew I had done extremely well but when the results came, I was overjoyed. I had stood first, not only in the college but in the whole university as well! It was unbelievable. When I went to pay my respects to Professor Murthy and asked him how I could repay him, he was furious and told me that he was in this profession because of his passion for teaching, not for the money.

This incident taught me humility and how much love and compassion a teacher can have for his/her student. Here was a man, financially well-off, who had no need to even take up teaching, let alone take extra classes for a student. I was ready to give up, accepting that there was no future, when, all of a sudden, help came in the form of Professor Murthy, and the tables were turned. This taught me that nothing is impossible in life, if we are resilient. Resilience helped me overcome a series of setbacks that could have finished my career and crushed my dreams. It was my teacher's commitment and belief in me that inspired me to work doubly hard—put in more hours than I normally would, just like the poem 'The Ladder of St. Augustine' by Henry Wadsworth Longfellow, teaches us:

The heights by great men reached and kept
    Were not attained by sudden flight,
But they, while their companions slept,
    Were toiling upward in the night.

Standing on what too long we bore
    With shoulders bent and downcast eyes,
We may discern—unseen before—
    A path to higher destinies.

I believed that if I kept studying into the night while my classmates slept, I would be able to match up to them and, eventually, my belief reigned. And it was Prof. Murthy who helped me build the muscle of resilience. But even after I did well in the exams, getting into the medical college wasn't easy.

After limited preparation, I appeared for the JIPMER (Jawaharlal Institute of Postgraduate Medical Education and Research) entrance exam at Puducherry (then known as Pondicherry). However, despite attaining the second rank in the all-India exam, my father persuaded me to give up my seat. His reasoning was that as I was the university topper, I would definitely get a seat in one of the government medical colleges in Chennai. He said, 'How can you work with me on diabetes during your undergraduate medical course if you are studying in another city?' This logic made sense. For the same reason, he persuaded me to not appear for the interview round of St John's Medical College in Bangalore (now Bengaluru). Because of his deep love for his alma mater, he compelled me to fill in 'Stanley Medical College' as all three choices for government medical colleges that one is allowed to opt for in the application form. But when the results came, I was chosen for the Madras Medical College, and that was where I eventually went.

As we go through life, we begin to realize that it is never a bed of roses. There are always ups and downs. Out of the blue, misfortune can fall upon us. This can occur in many ways. A person in the absolute pink of health, an athlete who is always full of energy, is suddenly hit by a truck. From that moment onwards, his life changes completely and perhaps can never be the same again. A businessman is raking in millions when, suddenly, there is an unexpected slump in his business and he goes bankrupt. You are happily married to the love of your life and life could not be sweeter, when, suddenly, he or she dies of a strange illness. It is natural for people to be heartbroken and face depression for a while after the loss of a loved one, or the loss of a job, or after losing a game, or not topping an examination. All these are bound to happen at some time or the other, to all of us. Those who are resilient recover quickly from their setback and are able to adjust to the misfortune or change that has occurred in their life. Others are not able to accept it for months, years or even decades after the incident has occurred. For somebody to be successful in life, resilience is extremely important.

The lives of many heroes teach us how resilient they are. During my childhood, I was inspired by the life story of Abebe Bikila, a relatively unknown Ethiopian long-distance runner who shot to fame after winning the marathon in the Rome and Tokyo Olympic games. He was the first person to win the Olympic marathon twice. Shortly after, Bikila had a serious car accident which rendered him a quadriplegic. He completely lost all movement in his body from his neck downwards. After several months of physiotherapy, his hands recovered but he still remained paraplegic, that is, paralysed below the waist, and was thereafter confined to a wheelchair for the rest of his life. Sitting in his wheelchair, Bikila now took up a new sport—archery—and he went on to become an archery champion. Bikila's story is an unparalleled inspiration to millions of people who may be differently abled, either from birth or due to an accident or an illness later in life. This is where the power of resilience kicks in. We should always remember that nobody, and nothing, in this world, can, or should, put us down.

In my life, the best example of resilience I see is my wife. Rema was just reaching the peak of her career as an ophthalmologist and a specialist in retinal diseases when she was diagnosed with breast cancer. This was a huge blow, not only for her but for the whole family. The news came crashing down on us just when we were struggling to establish our practice and had huge loans to pay back. How Rema fought her breast cancer even when it was diagnosed at a fairly advanced stage, is a remarkable story.

The first few months went in undergoing various treatments, including surgery, chemotherapy and radiotherapy. But during this time, Rema continued to work from home. It was during this difficult period that she wrote her PhD thesis and eventually became the first ophthalmologist in India to obtain a PhD degree. Although a clinician, Rema did basic research on the biochemistry of diabetic eye disease, which was most unusual for an ophthalmologist.

Not only was she able to get back to work soon, she actually took on more responsibilities. She started several new research projects in diabetic retinopathy and even established a separate building for treatment and research on diabetic eye diseases, probably the only one of its kind in the world. As the managing director of our hospital, she managed the entire administration and proved to be an able administrator who won the love and affection of the entire team. Under her able leadership, the DMDSC brand grew and we started establishing branches of our centre in different parts of the country. Rema was personally involved in the planning and execution of these various projects. She also published a large number of research papers (well over a hundred), which is unique, considering that she worked in the narrow field of diabetic eye diseases. Throughout her life, she has donned multiple hats—clinical responsibilities, research, teaching and administration, in addition to fulfilling all her family and social responsibilities.

Everything went well for about thirteen years. But in 2007, during a routine annual check-up, it was detected that Rema's cancer had returned and spread to the lungs. This meant that she had to undergo several rounds of chemotherapy and other hormonal treatments, while continuing to do her multivarious activities. The disease, then, would briefly go into remission, only to come back later with renewed aggression. This went on for over four years. By the end of 2010, it was becoming clear that Rema was slowly losing the battle against cancer. Never one to get depressed, she rapidly made plans for the future and her succession both on the administrative side as well as in her chosen speciality. She trained several ophthalmologists who, to this day, continue the dedicated and specialized work in the field that she established.

By the beginning of 2011, Rema's movements were beginning to get restricted and she ultimately became bedridden. It was at this time that her resilience really amazed me. One of her research students who was working on diabetic retinopathy was completing her PhD. She had written her thesis but it had to be corrected before submitting to the university. Confined to her bed, Rema took on the onerous task of going through the entire PhD thesis. She meticulously made corrections and gave several suggestions for improvement. At one point, I offered to help, but she politely declined, saying, 'Mohan, please allow me to complete all my duties. It is *my* duty to help my student. Let me do it myself.'

She also took special care to train several people, including her sister, Rekha, and daughter, Anjana, in running the administrative affairs of the centre in her absence. By March 2011, she had completed all the tasks she had assigned to herself and passed away with dignity and poise. It was a touching and emotionally moving scene. Her mother and sister, our daughter and I were all holding her hand when she smiled for the last time and then passed into infinity. We could almost see her merge with the divine.

It is amazing that someone who is in the last stages of her life was able to contribute so much to everything and everyone around her. Rema's story is undoubtedly the best example of resilience that I have seen in my life, and it taught me the vital lesson that it is never too late to serve others, even if one is on one's deathbed.

7

Early Lessons in Empathy

Empathy is a quality of character that can change the world.

—Barack Obama, forty-fourth President of the United States

My primary school, St Kevin's, where I studied up to the fourth standard, was literally opposite my home in Royapuram, and I have many memories from my time there. But there are a couple of incidents etched in my mind. One evening, while studying in the third standard, I was getting ready to go home when something smacked my head and I started bleeding profusely. I turned around and noticed that one of my classmates had thrown a stone. He was aiming for the tamarind tree but it hit me instead. The teachers came running and I was rushed to the closest hospital, which happened to be my father's. I needed four stitches in order to stop the bleeding and close the wound. The repercussions were equally dramatic—not only was the boy punished, but to our surprise, the next day, the Mother Superior ordered that the tree be cut down. My father tried to talk to her and the other nuns to pacify them, saying that it was only an accident and that there was no need to cut the tree. But the Mother Superior was firm. As long as the tree stood there, she felt more boys would be tempted to throw stones, and she did not want such incidents taking place in her school.

I was no stranger to death and destruction. In some ways, life had been preparing me to be a doctor since I was born. When I was nine years old, I witnessed an old compound wall fall in my school. At lunchtime, several children were sitting very close to the wall, enjoying their meals, when, suddenly, it collapsed. From its external appearance, one would never have thought that the wall was this weak, but it was. Several children were trapped under the debris, and at least three or four children died in this tragic accident. I remember the bodies of the children, covered in mud, being taken to the hospital. It is a sight that haunted me for years.

From St Kevin's, I moved to St Mary's High School, where I was considered an ideal student. I consistently focused on academics and was motivated by awards and appreciation. Unfortunately, in those days, the school didn't award prizes to those who excelled in academics. It was a huge grouse for me—that even after I broke the school record by scoring the highest number of marks in the final school-leaving examinations and even received a state rank, I wasn't awarded a certificate or trophy. Sometimes a job well done is rewarding enough, but I believe in appreciating hard work, and so I recently instituted a Dr V. Mohan Gold Medal, with a certificate and cash prize for the best outgoing student of St Mary's High School.

However, St Mary's High School, or more specifically, Father Gregory Devarajan, the then principal of the school, made up for everything during its 175th anniversary celebrations held in 2014. The former President of India, the late Dr A.P.J. Abdul Kalam, was the chief guest, and I was honoured by my school for topping my class and setting a record that stood for three decades.

I might have been a sincere and exemplary student at St Mary's, where all the teachers and particularly the principal doted on me.

But there is an incident that I distinctly remember which cannot really counted as an achievement. When I was in the eighth standard, Mr Edmonds was our fiercely strict mathematics teacher and a complete no-nonsense man. One day, we students were waiting for Mr Edmonds to arrive, and I was sitting next to my friend and checking my maths homework against his. The first five problems were correct, and then my friend asked me about the sixth one. 'What sixth problem?' I asked, confused. 'There were only five.' There were six, he corrected me, and turned the page to show where the last problem was lurking. I had failed to turn the page and knew that my honest mistake would cost me dearly.

I knew that Mr Edmonds would arrive over the next few minutes, and that if anyone had missed solving a problem, he would definitely be punished. My only option was to quickly copy the answer from my friend. I took his notebook and was so engrossed in copying the steps that I did not notice the teacher coming in and standing behind me. Nor did I notice the eerie silence which enveloped the classroom. I had just finished copying everything and looked up to find, peering over my shoulder and watching me copying, Mr Edmonds. I had been caught red-handed!

'You are *copying*!' he yelled. His piercing voice filled the classroom and shook every single student into sitting stiller than usual. 'Sir,' I stammered, when he continued to scream. 'You are *copying*!' he yelled again. I gulped with difficulty, barely mouthing *yes*.

Infuriated, he asked me to get out of the classroom. So here was the top student of the class, evicted from it as punishment. Head hanging low, I stood in the veranda; about five minutes later, the principal, Father G.P. Whyte, walked by. He wondered what I was doing outside class. At that point I broke down and tried to explain my predicament to him: that I didn't have any intention to copy the answer. He brushed aside my explanations with a wave of his hand and, with a genuine, fatherly smile, asked me to follow him.

I was even more terrified because I thought I was going to get a scolding from Father. But when we reached his room, he asked if I would drink coffee or tea. I was taken aback and told him some coffee would be nice. Father brought me the coffee and asked me to relax. 'This is not the end of the world,' he said. 'I know you would not have done anything wrong on purpose. You relax in my room for now, and when the bell rings, you can go back to class.' Then he asked me whether I would like to listen to some music and proceeded to play some soft tunes for me. I was utterly confused, unable to understand what Father was up to, but I did as he said, and in no time, I was calm, my nerves soothed and the incident already history. In that moment I became Father's biggest fan, his most ardent admirer. He had trusted me and taught me a lesson I would carry for life. I would go on to use the same principles of trust, empathy and encouragement when I built my own institution— remembering at every step the kindness of my school principal, Father Whyte.

8

Dare to Dream Big

Whatever you do, or dream you can, begin it. Boldness has genius and power and magic in it.

—Johann Wolfgang von Goethe,
pre-eminent German writer and statesman

After I completed my high school at St Mary's Anglo-Indian High School, Chennai, I went to meet Father G.P. Whyte again, for the dual purpose of getting some advice regarding my future and also to get his autograph in my autograph book. The words which Father Whyte wrote for me had a profound influence on me, as he was someone whom I looked up to very much. He wrote: *Life is for those who dare.*

As a fifteen-year-old, I could not understand the depth of his statement. It was several years later, when I went through my autograph book again, that the profundity of Father Whyte's statement hit me. Yes life *is* indeed for those who dare. The meek and the timid will fall by the wayside, and it is the bold and those who dare to dream big who really make it in life. I would go as far as to say that daring to dream big is the very blueprint of success, particularly for an entrepreneur. But it holds true equally true for any other profession.

When I joined the medical college, I developed an intense passion for research. But my journey was not one without obstacles. I learnt the basics of clinical research while working with my father. When I joined him, his clinic was basically an old rented building that housed the outpatient and inpatient departments. The building also had a dilapidated garage. Like many start-ups with humble beginnings, our story, too, began in a garage. We bought a few cages of rats and mice and converted this space into a research lab. We hired a retired professor of biochemistry to run the lab. I was in my second year of medical college and worked closely with this professor, conducting various research experiments. We began by testing the metabolic effects of alcohol in mice and rats and also worked on figuring out the best way to measure blood glucose levels, as the enzymatic methods for glucose estimation were just being introduced at the time.

When I moved into my third year of medicine, my classmates and I asked our pharmacology professor, Professor Lalitha Kameswaran, for permission to carry out research during our summer holidays. I was inspired by Frederick Banting and Charles Best's famous dog experiments at the University of Toronto, Canada, which ultimately led to the discovery of insulin and the Nobel Prize for Medicine. Every day, I dreamt of a cure for diabetes, and I knew that immersing myself in research was the way to do it.

In the summer of 1973, we managed to conduct experimental research at Madras Medical College. I worked on diabetes, carrying out preclinical trials of a combination of two groups of anti-diabetic drugs—sulphonylureas (which stimulate a release of insulin from the pancreas) and biguanides (which make insulin more effective by reducing insulin resistance). They showed that the use of these two agents together had a synergistic effect in bringing down blood glucose levels. This is standard treatment for diabetes now but was relatively unknown at that time. I later started a clinical trial on patients with diabetes along with my father, which again showed us that using the two drugs in combination helped achieve better results with fewer side effects. These findings led to the very popular use of combination therapy of oral anti-diabetic drugs in India and indeed it is fair to say that, today, India is a world leader in the fixed-dose combination of anti-diabetic drugs.

Conducting research, however, was not easy in those days. Very little funding was available and journals were in short supply. In the early 1970s, there were few computers in India and certainly none in the hospitals. There was no Internet, and therefore no PubMed (the portal published by the National Institutes of Health which lists all journal articles) or Google. If one wanted journal references, one would have to visit several libraries as no single library stocked all the journals. I therefore made it a weekly habit to visit the British Council and the United States Information Services library attached to the American Consulate in Chennai, to read the latest issues of medical journals like the *Lancet*, the *British Medical Journal* and the *New England Journal of Medicine*. Luckily, photocopying machines had arrived on the scene by then and I would make copies of the articles I needed for my research.

Occasionally, when I could not find some urgently needed journals, I would make a trip to Delhi, to the National Medical Library, and spend a day or two there perusing the various journals, making a list of the references I needed and paying for them all in advance. They would then be photocopied and sent to me by surface mail. The articles would typically arrive several weeks later in Chennai. Today, when researchers and medical students tell me they find it very difficult to do research in a developing country like India due to limited facilities, I smile and look back at the time when we started our research with absolutely no resources whatsoever. Today, one just has to use Google or PubMed and, right on our smartphones, we can get whatever references we want. If one really wants to, one can find enough resources, funds and support to pursue their dreams.

To me, however, the challenge I faced in those days was an important lesson in life. It taught me to work hard, focus on what I wanted and follow my passion. These traits have stood me in good stead all my life.

Meanwhile, our work had started receiving recognition within a few years, not only nationally but also internationally. By the end of my MBBS course in 1976, our centre was recognized as a Scientific and Industrial Research Organization by the Government of India. This gave us the opportunity to apply for research grants. In those days, a private medical institution applying for, and successfully obtaining, a research grant was unheard of. Research was considered the domain of medical colleges, universities and government departments. People heading government departments wondered why doctors like me in private practice would even *want* to do research. 'What is your motive?' they asked. Telling them it was my *passion* was not considered a satisfactory reply. We persisted despite all the difficulties and, slowly, the research work we did, and our publications, began to get wider acceptance.

After Rema and I returned from the UK and Germany in 1986, I was very keen to build a full-fledged research centre in a separate building. My father, however, was sceptical, as he felt that establishing and maintaining a research institute, entirely with private funds, was just not feasible. After I left my father's practice in 1991 and started my own, the first five years went in building up the new clinical facilities. However, in my subconscious mind, I nurtured a dream of establishing a research centre of my own, and my passion for this kept building. In 1996, I finally took the plunge and hired our first research officer, and converted a small room in our hospital into a research laboratory. Thus was born, with one staff member and in one small room, what has eventually come to be known, nationally and internationally, as the Madras Diabetes Research Foundation. With the appointment of a full-time research officer, research work rapidly progressed at MDRF. We soon hired other staff members and started a clinical trials department, a cell and molecular biology department for doing basic science research and a genomics lab. We started merging one room after another in the hospital into the research lab, much to the consternation of our clinical colleagues and administrators. It soon became quite obvious that we had to build a separate research facility. Next door to our hospital, there was a piece of vacant land. I dreamt of putting up a separate building for research there. Very soon, this dream came true. We managed to purchase the land with the help of a friend but then soon faced the next problem. How do we get the money to erect the research building?

Around this time, a young man, Mr Surya Jhunjhunwala, came to see me. He introduced himself as an industrialist, with offices in Singapore and Hong Kong. His late father had diabetes, and had stipulated in his will that a sizable sum of money be donated to establish a research centre for diabetes, anywhere in the world. Surya had travelled to a few countries before coming to India to see me. On hearing our plan for the expansion of the research centre, and after consulting his family, he offered to donate the money required. Things moved swiftly and, within a short time, a separate building for the Madras Diabetes Research Foundation was established, next to our hospital campus. We named it the 'S.S. Jhunjhunwala Research Centre', after the donor, the late Sri S.S. Jhunjhunwala.

However, at the time of the inauguration of the building, I was surprised when senior scientists, administrators and visionary doctors, who had built institutions in the past, told me, like my father had earlier, that this would not be a sustainable venture. They even suggested that we convert half of the new building into clinical departments, by adding additional inpatient beds for the hospital, because that would give us a good and steady source of income.

Contrary to their fears, over the next few years, MDRF continued to expand and soon we were looking for additional space. It then came to our knowledge that there was a large piece of land available in the Women's Biotech Park at Siruseri, on the outskirts of Chennai, and that women entrepreneurs with a scientific background could apply to get land on a long lease to set up research institutes or biotech ventures. Rema applied for this opportunity, and we drew up an ambitious plan to build a centre of excellence for diabetes research at Siruseri. Prof. M.S. Swaminathan, the legendary agricultural scientist, was in charge of the project at that time. He was impressed with our plan which was quickly approved, and we were allotted 6.5 acres of land in the Biotech Park at Siruseri. With the support of friends and well-wishers, MDRF established a facility spanning 32,000 square feet, exclusively for diabetes research, with separate departments for epidemiology, cell and molecular biology, vascular biology, advanced research biochemistry and genomics, as well as tissue culture labs, food and nutrition research labs, statistics and data management and a central instrument and biorepository facility. MDRF has now grown to become the largest diabetes research centre in India. And it is humbling to note that all this started with the dream of establishing a research centre for diabetes. From a small room in a hospital with one staff member, it grew to where we are now. I am convinced that if one has the courage to dream and follow one's passion, a mystical, powerful and universal force appears to fuel these dreams and ultimately turn them into reality.

However, we need the support of the right people, at the right time, in order to achieve our dreams. Once, I was on a short flight from Bangalore to Chennai, and sitting next to me was Dr Kallam Anji Reddy, chairman of Dr Reddy's Laboratories. Dr Reddy was a self-made man. After working for a government pharma company for a few years, he started his own. This venture grew exponentially to become the world-renowned Dr Reddy's Laboratories, one of India's largest pharma companies. What set apart Dr Reddy was not just the industries he established but also his passion for research. He was a scientist and a technocrat and had a dream of producing a new Indian-made drug for diabetes and metabolic disorders. It was my first meeting with Dr Reddy, but by the end of that thirty-minute flight, we felt we had known each other for years.

Dr Reddy was a great source of support to me and our research foundation. I was also privileged to be his physician and diabetologist. Like Dr Reddy, many other friends extended their support to us in all our activities. If not for them, we would never have made it this far in life.

9

Passion: The Key to Success

I would rather die of passion than of boredom.

—Émile Zola, French novelist, critic and political activist

Truly speaking, my father is my 'medical' guru; he was a pioneer in diabetology, and my initial interest in the disease and its research came about because of him. As I began working with him, even in the 1970s, I could see diabetes progressing at an alarming rate among Indians, warning those paying attention of an imminent epidemic. The more I read about diabetes, the more it consumed me, to a point that it was no longer a passion but an obsession.

My father began to notice that I was taking an extraordinary interest in diabetes for a medical student. He was happy but also fearful that I was neglecting the other subjects. Hence, he set down certain conditions with regard to how and what I could study. If I wanted to spend more time reading about diabetes, he said, it had to be done after studying for my university examinations. So, at midnight, I would shut my university textbooks to open journals that published articles about diabetes. The many nights I spent reading and researching about diabetes taught me an important lesson: when one is passionate about something, one has extraordinary energy; a person then never feels tired and is willing to sacrifice anything, including sleep, in order to fulfil that passion.

I would come home tired after a hard day at the office and, just when I thought I was exhausted and ready to sleep, I would remember an urgent research paper waiting for my attention. Instantly, my tiredness would vanish and I would feel a fresh burst of energy that would keep me going for the next few hours.

It was 2009. I was on an international flight from Chennai to Singapore. It was 2 a.m. and everyone on the flight was asleep. I was reading a research paper, when an idea struck me. It came at me with such force that I immediately took out a few loose sheets of paper from my bag and began writing. I must have been working away for a long time, because I didn't notice that an air hostess was standing behind me, peering down my shoulder.

I was startled to see her standing behind me. 'What are you working on so seriously that stops you from sleeping at this time, sir?' she asked. 'I was trying to complete an important research paper,' I said. 'I wanted to finish it before I forget the idea, and once I got into the mood, I didn't notice the time.' 'Almost everyone catches up on missed sleep on flights. I have never seen anyone work as hard as you,' she said, smiling. But to me, it was nothing unusual. Just like how musicians or writers can be completely lost and immersed in their art, so are people like me. This is what passion is all about: it gives you a sense of purpose in life; it is an extension of you and constitutes a realization that something is far more important than life's everydayness.

After I completed my PhD, one of my teachers, Prof. S.P. Thiagarajan, persuaded me to work for the Doctor of Science (DSc) degree, which is considered the highest research degree in India. To receive this degree, one has to submit a thesis consisting of a series of research publications on a specific topic. I had enough publications but still needed to knit them together and include some additional material. The problem was that I could not find any time to work on my DSc thesis.

Once I found out that I had to travel from Chennai to Delhi four times in one month, I realized that each flight would give me two and a half hours of uninterrupted time. I decided to write the entire DSc thesis while on these eight flights, and at the end of the month, my DSc thesis was ready for submission. I have heard similar stories from people in different fields—people who manage to achieve extraordinary feats in a limited time because they were passionate and driven about what they were doing.

And this is why, among the various traits needed for success, I would place passion on top of the list. If you have passion, a fire in the belly, zest, zeal, fervour, enthusiasm or simply a strong interest in something, you will sacrifice anything for it. One can acquire a lot of skill, knowledge or experience. But unless one has passion, one can rarely achieve one's goals.

Sachin Tendulkar, the great cricketing legend of India, is often described as the 'god of cricket' by Indians and is admired by people all over the world for his unparalleled batting talent. His passion for cricket was ignited when he was a child and received a cricket bat as a birthday present. With the support of his brother and other family members, he started going for cricket coaching when he was in school. By the time he was a teenager, he was already playing test cricket for India. Sachin dreamt about cricket day and night. His passion was so intense that cricket became his life. He went on to set several world records, including hitting a hundred centuries, an unbelievable, almost superhuman, achievement! Shortly after achieving that historic milestone, he was asked by a reporter whether he was finally ready to retire. Sachin instantly replied with his characteristic smile on his face, 'No. I will continue to play the game as long as my passion for the game remains.'

When I had the opportunity to meet Sachin and chat with him, I was greatly impressed by his love for cricket and his total commitment to the game. But it also led me to think: Can such an unbridled passion be induced?

Perhaps not. It is not possible to inject passion into anyone. It's intrinsic, within you. God gives different people different passions, different abilities and different dreams. There is a common mistake that parents make, of trying to mould their children into something that they (the parents) wish for. There are many instances of people changing their careers either after they completed a course that they were forced to take up, or worse, after continuing in that field for many years, only to realize that it was not making them happy. But if a person is passionate, he or she would go far beyond the call of duty. Thereafter, time and place do not matter any more. What would have otherwise been a strictly nine-to-five job now has no time limits. They would willingly come to work early and stay well beyond their official office hours. They are also constantly pursuing their passion at every waking moment. If it is music that they are interested in, they would be willing to spend hours practising on their guitar or piano. The more they work on it, the happier they become.

Passion is also infectious as it results in better teamwork and automatically makes the person with passion a leader. In fact, one of the greatest qualities or attributes of a leader is that they are so passionate about what they do that they motivate others to work and make it an enjoyable experience for all. The passionate individual's boundless energy leads to hard work, which is all managed in an atmosphere of comradeship, combined with a lot of fun, because of which success is ensured.

10

By Sharing Your Knowledge, You Also Grow in the Process

Thousands of candles can be lighted from a single candle, and the life of the original candle will not be shortened. Happiness never decreases by being shared.

—Gautama Buddha, the founder of Buddhism

Early in my career, I realized that as an individual doctor, I could only see a limited number of patients, say, a maximum of twenty or twenty-five per day. This meant that in a lifetime I would have been able to touch the lives of a few thousand people. I then thought: *What if I trained my students to follow the same treatment methods and we all worked as a team?* We could obviously multiply the impact we make manyfold and improve the lives of millions of people.

Therefore, in 1981, when I completed my postgraduate training in medicine and joined my father as a full-time consultant, I told my father, 'Dad, I think it is time we started capacity-building activities in India to tackle the looming diabetes epidemic. We have to train doctors to treat diabetes using the standardized protocols that we have developed over the years. As we were not attached to a medical college, one way we could do this was by starting a fellowship in diabetes. That same year, we started the first 'fellowship in diabetes' programme in India, with three students.

When my wife, Rema, and I started Dr Mohan's Diabetes Specialities Centre in 1991, it occurred to us that if we wanted to see our dream of being able to treat diabetes on a national level fulfilled, it would mean that we would first have to create an entire ecosystem for diabetes treatment, which would consist of training not only thousands of doctors but also nurses, dieticians, educators and technicians.

We first expanded the fellowship programme, and currently we have about twenty doctors who are trained as fellows in diabetes every year. Over the past forty years, we have trained several hundred doctors from all over the country, many of whom have gone ahead to set up their own, very successful, diabetes clinics. The Tamil Nadu Dr MGR Medical University later permitted us to start a postdoctoral fellowship in the diabetes course for doctors who already had a postgraduate degree, i.e. an MD in internal (general) medicine. Along with this, we started several other courses at our centre, like a postgraduate diploma in diabetes education and a fellowship in diabetic eye diseases, to fulfil our vision of training in allied specialities around diabetology.

But these initiatives were all 'in-house programmes', where the students had to study full-time, and the numbers were still relatively small. I knew that if we wanted to reach the whole country and train doctors to treat millions of people with diabetes, we would have to scale up these efforts. To take on such an ambitious project, we would have to collaborate with several doctors, specifically, diabetologists and endocrinologists across the country.

Around this time, I got a call from the Public Health Foundation of India (PHFI), New Delhi, demonstrating an interest in helping us with a national programme to cover the country. The PHFI had the capacity to reach all over India because of its extensive network, and I was excited about the possibilities the collaboration would bring. When we started working with the PHFI, we made plans of converting our existing diabetes course material into a format that could be applied on a larger scale without requiring doctors to spend a year or two full-time at our centre. My son-in-law, Dr Ranjit Unnikrishnan, evinced keen interest in taking up this challenge and preparing the course material. Several top diabetologists and endocrinologists also volunteered their time and expertise. A pharma company offered an unrestricted grant to support the programme. This partnership led to the development of a large-scale programme to train physicians in diabetes, called the Certificate Course in Evidence-Based Diabetes Mellitus (CCEBDM).

Next came the planning stage. With India's top diabetologists and endocrinologists now on board, the popularity of the course went up immensely. But a thought kept troubling me: even with a twelve-to-fifteen-member-large faculty, consisting of very senior experts, it would be impossible to scale the project up to the level I had imagined: to create a complete ecosystem for diabetes prevention and control in India. Therefore, the next step was to identify regional faculty who would be able to conduct these classes in their respective cities.

In the following months, we were able to identify over a hundred regional faculty members comprising diabetologists and endocrinologists across the country who expressed their willingness and keen interest in participating in the project. We then drew up a plan setting out how the CCEBDM would be conducted. The national faculty, we decided, would finalize the course content and would also train the regional faculty.

Each of the regional faculty members would then train a small group of ten to twelve doctors in their respective cities or towns. This would have the desired 'multiplier effect' and markedly increase the number of doctors trained.

The main attractions were that the course had a low fee, a detailed twelve-module structure, and was deliberately scheduled over the weekends to enable maximum participation by doctors without disrupting their work schedule or their practice.

There were a number of roadblocks, too. A few of the regional faculty were extremely committed, while others showed merely a lukewarm interest. Similarly, while most of the national faculty were deeply engaged in the programme, one or two of them were unable to devote enough time. But the most important aspect was the support provided by the PHFI. They did all the groundwork and deputed a large number of staff members to oversee the quality of the programme. They would also regularly organize national and regional faculty-training workshops and also periodically assess the quality of the programmes by conducting surprise visits to the centres.

Over six cycles of the CCEBDM, 13,300 physicians have been successfully trained in diabetes. Even if we assume that each physician would go on to treat a conservative figure of a thousand patients with diabetes, the lives of over 13 million Indians with diabetes would have been touched and their quality of care improved dramatically. We were, naturally, pleased with the results obtained due to a multiple-level collaboration on a national scale, the likes of which had never been attempted before.

The CCEBDM has also been adopted by around eight state governments in India, with many more in the pipeline. On an international level, the health ministries of the governments of Rwanda, Myanmar, Bangladesh, Afghanistan and Nepal have adopted the course as well. What started as a small programme to train physicians in diabetes care has now become a huge national and international capacity-building programme in the field of diabetes—the largest of its kind in the world.

The CCEBDM was also selected as an 'Innovation Model of Education' by the Government of India at their Innovation Summit in 2017, and also received recognition from the South Asian Federation of Endocrine Societies. We did not stop there, however. Similar certificate courses were later started, in conjunction with the PHFI, for gestational diabetes mellitus, diabetic retinopathy and cardiovascular disease, among others. But the CCEBDM is the biggest example of what transpires if there is a willingness to share knowledge. Many fellow diabetologists and doctors from all over India regularly tell me that they have never seen a course create such so much interest, passion and unity among the medical community. It is perhaps one of our greatest achievements that the CCEBDM turned out to be one of the biggest success stories in skilling and capacity building in the field of medicine in India.

But the work had to continue and there was no shortage of ideas. During my visits abroad, I had observed how trained diabetes educators in the US, the UK, Germany, Canada, Australia and other developed countries would help physicians in their diabetes clinics by reaching out to patients and providing them with valuable diabetes education—most importantly, spending time with patients, something that the overburdened physicians could ill afford. Inspired by the success of various PHFI courses for doctors, we started collaborating with other organizations to start courses for paramedical personnel as well. A National Diabetes Educator Program (NDEP) was initiated with the help of the Indian Diabetes Educators Association, the support of Dr Shashank Joshi and Shilpa Joshi, my colleagues in Mumbai, and an unrestricted educational grant by a pharma company. The aim was to train diabetes educators across the country. The NDEP programme helped fill this void. Following a model similar to what we had adopted for the CCEBDM course, we trained ninety-seven regional faculty members comprising diabetologists and endocrinologists, each of whom trained ten to twenty diabetes educators. Within a few years, we were able to develop a cadre of over 13,000 diabetes educators in India. A journal specifically meant for diabetes educators was also established. The NDEP became one of the largest diabetes-educators' courses outside developed countries like the US or the UK.

The idea of sharing knowledge is robust and multifold, and I began to identify multiple gaps that could be filled with innovation. Nurses, for instance, are traditionally trained to perform their general nursing duties. However, with increasing specialization, nurses are now trained in different specialized fields, for instance, cardiothoracic, neurological or psychiatric nursing. The concept of 'diabetes nurse educators' was unheard of in India, although it is very popular in the West. Seeing this as a great opportunity, in collaboration with Deakin University, Melbourne, Australia, a Deakin–DMDEA course for diabetes nurse educators was developed by us. This turned out to be a huge success and several batches of diabetes nurse educators have now completed and obtained their diplomas from Deakin University. A new sub-speciality of diabetes nurse educators has been born in India!

And so my dream of building a complete ecosystem for diabetes care, research, prevention and control was fulfilled. What pleases me the most is that this has helped touch the lives of millions of people both in India and abroad. Indeed, it is extremely gratifying to note that in doing so we have incidentally also fulfilled our mandate as a World Health Organization collaborating centre for the prevention and control of NCDs and as an International Diabetes Federation (IDF) Centre of Excellence in Diabetes Education.

11

Failure Is Never Final

The only man who never makes a mistake is the man who never does anything.

—Theodore Roosevelt,
twenty-sixth President of the United States

I am often asked whether life has been a streak of continuous successes for me or have I also tasted failure. Life has certainly not been bereft of challenges and I have experienced my fair share of setbacks and failures. In 1991, when we left the comfort of my father's centre, Rema and I had no clue about how to start a clinic of our own. As the reality of what we had done started to sink in, doubts started surfacing. We were guided by our unwavering vision and commitment, but no matter how we proceeded, setbacks crowded our way. Initially, we decided (in retrospect, rather foolishly) to immediately buy a piece of land with a building and start a full-fledged hospital for diabetes with outpatient and inpatient services. We located, what we thought at the time, was a suitable property in Mylapore, in the heart of Chennai. We signed an agreement with the owner, a lawyer, and paid him a substantial sum of money as an advance. This money wasn't ours but what we had borrowed from friends.

As the money wasn't sufficient, we also started applying for an additional loan to buy the property. A few months later, while the loan was being processed and the architect's plans were being drawn up, we received some shocking news. A legal notice, from the residents living on the same road as the property we had invested in, had arrived. It prohibited us from starting a clinic on their road. The main reason they cited was that the road was quite narrow and they feared that if a clinic came up there, there would be a marked increase in traffic on that road. This was indeed true, because the area at the time was classified as a residential area, and if we were to open a clinic there, it would require a reclassification of the zone. The bureaucratic process would prove to be cumbersome, if not impossible.

Rema and I knew none of this, nor had we been warned by our lawyer; we had naively ventured into this project in a hurry. We were now terrified at the prospect of the owner of the property refusing to return the advance by terming it a breach of contract. This, we feared, would lead to a protracted legal battle and would stall our prospects of starting a clinic, indefinitely. The fact that the owner was a lawyer himself didn't help matters.

However, our fears proved unfounded. After a couple of meetings with the neighbours (in the presence of the owner), it became quite clear that we would not be permitted to start our clinic there. We therefore volunteered to withdraw from the project and requested the owner to return the advance. And to our surprise, he promptly did so. With this, the first problem was solved. The next question was: How do we now proceed with the project?

This setback had made us rethink our plans. We realized that trying to *buy* a property was not a great idea due to the expensive real estate in Chennai. We therefore reworked our plans and decided to look for a *rented* premise which would not only be cheaper but would also make it much easier and quicker to start the project. While on the lookout for a new property to start our clinic, we came across a magnificent building on Royapettah High Road which seemed to suit our purpose. This was a commercial property on a wide road and hence there were no objections to the clinic. A setback had led to something much better. It was only because the residents had objected that we had pulled out of the Mylapore property. Had we gone ahead with the original project, we would have been stuck there indefinitely. Not only would there be no room for expansion, we would have also sunk a considerable amount of money into buying the property and hence it would have been difficult to sustain the clinic. With the rented building, our capital expenses for setting up the clinic were a fraction of the amount we had originally planned on spending. We were also able to start the project much faster, thus saving a considerable amount of time and money. In other words, the setback had brought us closer to success.

Today, when people see our centre's many branches, they remark that whatever I touch blossoms, and that I have never had to surmount pressing challenges or failures in life. While due diligence and the careful selection of the place where we want to start the branch, the location, the doctor, the team and the intensive training all ensure success in the majority of our ventures, there have been several instances of failures as well.

We started a branch in Goa, and it ran for a couple of years. But somehow we could not get enough patients to sustain it. And after two or three years, we decided to close down the Goa unit. We started a unit in Lucknow in Uttar Pradesh, a state where we were completely unknown. But we couldn't sustain it either. When the losses started mounting, we closed the centre. We also shut down another branch in Mangalore, one each in Delhi, Kochi and

Mysore, and also one in Chennai, which is our hometown, and our headquarters. All these were conscious decisions and the valuable lesson it taught us was that we should not spread ourselves too thin.

But a failure that crushed me most spectacularly and also taught me to focus on familiar territories and play my cards well was an effort to expand overseas. In 2012, a few of my patients had come to consult me from Muscat, Oman. They were proposing helping us set up a branch of our clinic in Muscat. The idea was very tempting. We had been expanding in India but had not opened any clinic outside our country. We soon found a local sponsor, received some investments from our patients and, after adding our own investments, we set up a separate company in Muscat. Things in Muscat move much slower than in India and hence it took us more than a year to set up the clinic. We hired two doctors and recruited other staff members. And, after further delays, we finally started our operations in Muscat in March 2014. I oversaw the project and continuously travelled between Chennai and Muscat, obtained a clinical registration to practise there and even saw patients at the clinic. Although we did see some partial success, it soon became obvious that operating in Muscat was a completely different ball game compared to running clinics in India.

To begin with, most patients in Muscat have insurance cover, and to enlist our company with the various insurance agencies was no easy task. The authorities, too, proved unresponsive, and all the processes and permissions took much longer than expected. Soon, the weeks turned into months and the months to years. We realized that we were steadily losing money, and the losses soon accumulated into huge sums of money. Several attempts to improve the business failed to bear fruit. Finally, a point of no return was reached and we had to take the painful decision of closing down our Muscat operations completely. Our first attempt at starting a diabetes clinic in a foreign land went up in smoke.

Over the years, we have had to shut down other centres in India as well, and each decision proves to be as painful as the last. When the team huddles together in meetings and discusses how certain centres aren't performing despite our best efforts, it is no more about one person's failure but the whole team's. There is nothing I hate more than seeing people walk out of the meeting room with long faces. Often, there is a sense of gloom and the team feels they have failed and not lived up to the expectations of the management or, worse, that the management let them down.

Was, then, the Muscat or Lucknow experience a sheer waste of time? The answer is *no*. Was the experiment worth it? Yes. If we hadn't experienced failure, we would have never learnt how to build better, more robust and more efficient centres that could withstand tough times. In other words, the very factors which led to our failure were the ones that would pave the way for our success in the future. If you study history, you will find that there are hundreds of people who have initially failed, before they eventually succeeded, and some of them eventually even made it really big in life. In fact, some of the most successful and famous people in the world have endured terrible failures at some point in their life. Some failed not once but repeatedly, and they failed repeatedly because they never stopped trying. If failure teaches you to stop trying, you're learning the wrong lesson. Failure is all about trying new things and doing them differently till you succeed.

In 2006, we were contemplating starting 'holistic' diabetes care, and the idea of starting an Ayurveda clinic at our Gopalapuram centre emerged. We bought rights to the franchise of a well-known Ayurveda clinic. But the project proved to be a miserable failure and we closed the clinic after two years. Patients told us quite bluntly that if they wanted Ayurvedic treatment, they would go elsewhere, to Ayurvedic hospitals or clinics, and not visit us.

Now, when I look back at all the times I have been rapped on the knuckles by failure, I also think about how resolute it has made me. The first lesson of course is to not cry over spilt milk; we have to spring back and look at failure in the eye, understand it deeply. And then beat it at its own game, for failure, as they say, is never final.

12

The Power of Grit

Only those who will risk going too far can possibly find out how far one can go.

—T.S. Eliot, American-English poet,
playwright, literary critic and editor

Angela Duckworth, in her excellent book entitled *Grit: The Power of Passion and Perseverance*, explains how passion and resilience are the secrets to success when present together with courage, or grit. She says that the main reason why some people give up halfway through any venture, while others persist in their efforts, is because of grit. It is the latter group of people who ultimately emerge as winners.

In recent times, one of the best examples of grit has been the cricketer Yuvraj Singh. Cricket fans still remember the match where Yuvraj Singh hit six sixes in a row at the ICC World T20 match against England, held at Kingsmead Stadium in Durban, South Africa, in 2007. Only a few cricketers in the world have been able to accomplish this feat.

I often show the video of this match to my students and juniors to teach them that achieving the impossible is possible, if we focus on the job at hand. Recently, when I travelled with Yuvraj Singh from Delhi to Chennai, I brought up the topic of his six sixes. I asked Yuvraj, 'Did you think you would be able to hit all six balls for sixes when you went in to bat that day?' Modest as always, Yuvraj replied, 'When one goes in to bat, no one knows how things will turn out. On some days, nothing goes wrong, and on others, you can get out for a duck.' Yuvraj said that it was partly his anger to prove a point to the Englishmen that probably made him achieve this feat. Shortly before Stuart Broad bowled that fateful over, Yuvraj had had an argument with Andrew Flintoff. However, it was not Flintoff but Stuart Broad who paid the price. 'When I hit the first two balls for sixes, I didn't think of this achievement at all. When I hit the third ball for a six, it dawned on me that I could try and continue this performance for the remaining three balls. When I hit the fourth six, there was a thundering applause from the crowd, and my heart was beginning to beat faster. When the fifth six happened, I told myself that I should try to complete the feat. I am happy I was able to achieve it.' One can only imagine the levels of concentration, focus and self-confidence that Yuvraj would had to have muster to achieve that near-impossible task. That's grit with a capital G!

Such examples are not limited to athletes or celebrities. My childhood friend Hari Baskaran grew up with several elder siblings. Very tragically, and inexplicably, all his siblings succumbed to cancer. In addition, his mother also died of cancer. With this background, I always marvelled at the positive attitude Hari has always maintained towards life. The sword of Damocles was always dangling over his head, but Hari continued to focus on keeping himself fit. After he retired at the age of sixty-four, he seriously took up cycling. And in January 2019, when he turned seventy, he decided to show the world that age is just a number. He undertook a long cyclothon journey from Chennai to Delhi. He did not take the shortest route to complete this journey. Instead, he zigzagged around India, going from Chennai to Bangalore, Mysore, Tumkur, Goa and Mumbai, before heading to Bhopal and finally reaching Delhi. He cycled over 3000 kilometres, resting at night and resuming the journey the following day. But his journey was not just about cycling. He met people living in old-age homes and treated them to motivational talks, showing them how age should not be a detriment to good health, or to achieving one's goals in life.

Hari continues to inspire me and has just published a book on celebrating active aging. Today, at the age of seventy-one, despite the fact that he has a 'myocardial bridge'—a heart condition which impairs his ability to do any form of strenuous activity from running to cycling—he has adopted a programme of alternate jogging and walking to keep his heart fit. Hari is planning to participate in a half marathon soon and later in a full marathon. I have heard of many gritty people but this is *grit extraordinaire*.

Hari staved off all illnesses with this positive outlook to life and the hard work that he put in through modifying his diet and physical activity. He also took to Buddhism and became a strong believer in spirituality. Through sheer grit, he was able to achieve things which those much younger than him have not been able to. Hari is a role model, an unsung hero and someone we must all look up to.

In my own life, I have been compelled to channel my inner gritty core, like any other hard-working medical student fuelled by sheer willpower and steel. During my compulsory rotating internship that all medical students are obliged to do before they graduate, for my medicine internship I was placed under an extremely knowledgeable but slightly eccentric professor who followed his own timings. He was known to give appointments to his patients at midnight and practise into the wee hours of the morning. This meant that the poor house surgeon (intern) on duty, in between seeing patients, writing case notes and getting investigations ready, also had to brief the boss at 1 a.m. The good thing about this grilling schedule was that it made us physically and mentally tough and got us ready to face any situation in life. The early years of medical college and practice were therefore a preparation in grit.

But if my medicine posting was tough, my surgical posting was even tougher. We worked under a renowned professor of surgery. While he was affable and often joked with the students, which resulted in his tremendous popularity, the house surgeons were terrified to work under him because he ran his unit with a military discipline. According to him, the house surgeon was in complete charge of the unit and was supposed to know every case or patient in the ward. Unlike my experience in the medicine department, where I only had to know the patients in the male or female ward, depending on where I was posted, in this surgical unit, one was expected to know all the cases in the male and female wards. This was a near-impossible task and most house surgeons found it difficult to cope with this expectation.

To make matters worse, the professor would tell us that he would meet us at the male general ward, and while we would be waiting there the next morning to present the case to him, he would go to the female general ward and start his rounds there. I later learnt from him that the reason he did this was to make sure that the house surgeon was alert at all times. When we confronted him one day, he explained to us the reason behind what seemed to us like an unnecessary mischief. 'What happens if you are the only doctor looking after the male and female wards, and you are in one ward and there is an emergency in the other? How would you handle this? This is the reason why I try to make you alert at all times,' he said.

These hardships trained us for a life of commitment and grit. We did make mistakes but, each time, our professors and seniors were there to guide us or correct us. I now realize that we were being taught lessons not just in medicine and surgery but also in grit. As Angela Duckworth says, 'To be gritty is to fall down seven times, and rise eight [times].'

13

Never Let People Discourage You

Successful people will always tell you that you can do something. It's the people who have never accomplished anything who will always discourage you from trying to achieve excellent things.

—Lou Holtz, former American
football player, coach and analyst

It was the year 1998. I was having dinner with a friend when I told him about the newest idea bubbling in my head: I wanted to conduct a mega show on diabetes for the public. I was inspired by the World Health Organization's newest and most powerful slogan which read, *Diabetes should go public.* This fired my imagination. I thought about it and realized that there are many huge expos organized for various purposes—real estate, jewellery, furniture, you name it. The thought then occurred to me: *Why not organize an expo on diabetes?* Nobody had done this earlier.

Before proceeding, however, I thought I should consult some friends. When I discussed this idea with one of my friends over dinner, he instantly ripped it apart. He felt that nobody would be interested in attending an expo on diabetes. He discouraged me with such surety and force, calling the idea 'boring', that I began to doubt it myself. He then gave me an alternate solution: 'There would be other expos in the city. Why don't you set up a small stall for diabetes at one of these events?' My big idea must have been unpalatable to him, but I had no desire to set up a stall in another expo. I tried to explain to him that my idea was not merely to set up one stall, but to have the whole expo on diabetes itself! He thought I was crazy and did not want to discuss the matter any more. I, too, decided to drop the project for some time.

But the idea kept coming back to me. Something kept egging me on to try, and I felt, with full sincerity and earnestness, that this would and could work, and that I should not give up so easily.

A couple of months later, I invited another friend home for dinner. Halfway through the meal, still terrified because of how the first friend I had approached had completely pooh-poohed the idea, I gathered courage and gingerly raised the topic of organizing an expo on diabetes. The man was thrilled! He said that it was a brilliant concept and even offered to help out with the project.

It thus transpired that in December 1998, we organized the first mega show on diabetes, called 'Diabetes 2000'. This acronym was used because the millennium year 2000 was just around the corner and we were showcasing diabetes in the next millennium. The event was a huge success, and something like this had not been witnessed anywhere. We had a huge crowd of people thronging to see what the first-ever diabetes exhibition was all about. The queues stretched half a mile outside the exhibition hall and the media covered the event live. Right next door, a furniture expo was being held. People had warned us that it would eclipse our event, but contrary to all expectations, there were far more people at our event than at the furniture expo. So much so that we had to seek police protection to control the crowd and the traffic. Word spread like wildfire after the first day, and on the subsequent days of the exhibition, we had to bring in extra security personnel to control the milling crowd. Diabetes 2000 had become a runaway success!

The event was then replicated several times, and each time it proved to be a staggering success, taking Chennai, Hyderabad, Madurai, Coimbatore and other cities in India by storm. If I had listened to the first friend I approached, perhaps Diabetes 2000 would have never seen the light of day, and if I hadn't found the courage to bring it up with my other friend, perhaps I would have been still mulling over an idea instead of taking it to fruition.

Quite often, it's our own mind that prevents us from recognizing and acting upon our brightest ideas or dreams. It's during those times that we have to recognize that what we need is a boost of self-confidence.

When Rema and I started our research foundation, we hired an outstanding researcher. It was thanks to her that we were able to rapidly scale up our research activities. She also quickly understood our research needs and was able to proactively plan, execute and publish research studies. I began to give her more and more responsibilities until she was responsible for conducting almost our entire research. One day, when we were in the thick of organizing a research seminar and had several ongoing projects due to a minor alteration, she suddenly decided to leave.

I was least prepared for this setback. I had got so used to depending on her as a scientist that I didn't know what to do. Work was in limbo and I was completely shattered. I wasn't sure how we would be able to carry on with research in her absence. Self-doubt began to creep in.

Days passed but my usual self-confidence didn't return. When Rema noticed this, she sat me down and, in her usual calm and composed manner, said, 'Mohan, just like you found her, we will find others. There will be somebody else who will be able to help you with our research. And in fact we will be increasing our research output in the years to come.' Initially, I found it difficult to believe her but I later realized that this was exactly what my inner voice was also telling me. Slowly, we were able to reassign that scientist's duties to other senior scientists in the organization and also hire some new staff members. I learned an important lesson through this incident: a lesson on decentralized empowerment, which allows multiple people in an organization to rise and grow, instead of having only one heroic leader.

But there was another learning point. When an inner voice communicates with you and tells you what to do, then you should listen to that voice and persist. Very often in life we meet naysayers, or are naysayers ourselves. We must be careful to avoid anything that dampens our spirits and enthusiasm. Conversely, there are people who exude optimism and positive energy. Just a few minutes in their presence results in our inner batteries getting fully charged and filling us with joy and enthusiasm. We should actively seek out and keep the company of such people and try to become like them ourselves.

14

Harness the Power of Collaboration

Collaboration is a key part of the success of any organization.

—Dinesh Paliwal, American business executive

In my early days, my research was limited to studying the case reports of patients, writing observations or doing clinical trials on newer molecules introduced by various pharmaceutical companies, as part of the drug-registration process in India. Soon, we started expanding our research by collecting data from multiple hospitals. This is where I first learnt the power of collaboration, because as you start collaborating with others, the quality and quantity of your research improves.

For the first twenty years of my research, I was mostly working with data collected on people with diabetes. I then realized a major lacuna in our studies. As our hospital dealt only with those who had diabetes, all our data only dealt with the various forms of diabetes. We had no data at all on people *without* diabetes. In other words, we had no idea what were the normal values for blood glucose levels, blood pressure, body weight, cholesterol or liver function tests for a wider demographic of people vis-à-vis different ages and genders. This was an undeniable limitation in our research studies as we could not compare the findings in our diabetic patients with normal people without diabetes. It was clear that broad, population-based epidemiological studies were required, and in 1998, we finally decided to step out of the comfort of our clinics and move into the community to do such research.

Initially, we kept it simple and started with 'convenience sampling' involving residential apartment owners who came forward to collaborate with us through common friends. We thus carried out the Chennai Urban Population Study (CUPS), our first epidemiology study focusing on lower- and middle-income groups. We studied a low-income settlement in T. Nagar and a middle-income housing colony in Thirumangalam. This study was the starting point of our journey in epidemiology, and although CUPS was a relatively small sample, with around 1500 participants, we managed to publish several papers from this study. The main finding from CUPS was that the prevalence rate of diabetes in the middle-income colony was almost double that of the low-income settlement. Although we were not surprised by the findings, it was the first intra-urban study of diabetes prevalence from India. However, the sample size of 1500 was far too small to draw meaningful conclusions, particularly in relation to the complications of diabetes. Moreover, the sample drawn was not representative of Chennai city; it was merely a 'convenience sample', which has much less scientific value, and the reviewers of the papers we wrote to promptly pointed this out to us.

At the time, there was no epidemiological data on diabetes complications in India or any other developing country. We realized that if we wanted to study the prevalence of the various complications of diabetes affecting the eyes, kidneys, nerves, heart and feet, we needed to study a much larger sample size. We then embarked on a larger epidemiological study, which would be completely representative of Chennai city. This became the well-known Chennai Urban Rural Epidemiological Study (CURES). Thanks to a large sample size of 26,000 and an excellent sampling frame, CURES helped answer several research questions and led to the publication of over 150 research papers in peer-reviewed journals. This is a record for a single research study in India—at least in the field of diabetes and metabolic diseases.

CURES fulfilled our ambition and provided valuable data on the prevalence of all diabetes complications for the first time in any developing country. It also provided the first instance of data on non-alcoholic fatty liver disease. Finally, it led to the development of a simple 'Indian diabetes risk' score that one could use to predict, with a high degree of accuracy, who was likely to develop diabetes within a community, even before a single drop of blood was drawn. This diabetes-risk score needed responses to just three questions relating to one's age, whether one's parents had diabetes and whether one did any physical activity. In addition, it required a simple waist measurement using a tailor's tape. It cost nothing and took just two minutes to administer the risk score. It could even be done online.

None of this was a one-person show. CURES was the result of a collaboration between MDRF, the Chennai Willingdon Corporate Foundation (a non-governmental organization), the Chennai Municipal Corporation and multiple residential colonies, and this took our research to another level.

Since then, the collaborations continued at a larger scale. One day, my daughter, Anju, who was doing her undergraduate medical course, approached me and said that she wanted to chat with me about something. We found some quiet time after dinner and I was reminded of my meeting with my father in the summer of 1968, which changed my life's course. She said, 'Can I be frank with you, Papa?' 'Of course,' I replied. 'Papa, all our research is so Chennai-centric. We are extrapolating the Chennai data to India. Chennai is not India, Papa. We have to think bigger.'

I was taken aback. 'What are you proposing we do?' I asked. Anju answered, 'We have to study the whole of India, Papa. We have to take up a truly national study of every state in India. Only then can we truly say that we have studied diabetes in India.'

When I heard this, my first thought was that she was crazy. India has a population of over 1.3 billion people, residing in twenty-eight states and eight union territories. The country boasts dozens of languages, thousands of dialects and tens of religions, with each state like a country in itself. But when Anju persisted, I bounced her presumably crazy idea off Prof. N.K. Ganguly, who, at the time, was the director general of the Indian Council of Medical Research (ICMR), during a casual meeting with him.

To my surprise, Prof. Ganguly loved the idea and asked us to make a formal presentation to the ICMR. And presto! Anju's idea was approved! Thus was born the ICMR–INDIAB (Indian Council of Medical Research–INdia DIABetes) study. Its primary objective was to study the prevalence of diabetes and prediabetes in India, with a sample size of 1,24,000 individuals—truly representative of India's 1.3-billion-strong population. This landmark study was made possible due to the generous support of the ICMR and the Department of Health Research, Government of India, as well as our numerous collaborators who served as the principal investigators in every state of India. The ICMR–INDIAB study also taught us to work in conjunction with the various state governments and health departments in India. The whole project has spanned over ten years to complete and, at the time of writing this book, is in its completion phase. To be fair to Anju, her passion for this study continues unabated to this day, with her taking full ownership of this near-impossible project.

The ICMR–INDIAB study can be described as a kaleidoscope representing India, and has taught us many things about our country's various cultural differences, habits and lifestyles. It has been one of the most enriching experiences of our lives, and I must appreciate my daughter's wisdom and foresight, and her ability to see much further than I could have ever done.

The most important lesson I have learned all through my career as a researcher is about the power of collaboration. I often hear from my colleagues that they are scared to collaborate with someone in research as they feel that they will be 'cheated' out of the glory due to them, or even worse, that their data will be stolen. My experience has taught me otherwise, and has in fact convinced me of the need for collaboration with multiple stakeholders for conducting successful research and taking things to the next level.

Examples of such successful collaboration include our experiences with Prof. K.M. Venkat Narayan (Venkat) of Emory University, Atlanta, in the US. Though we initially had no funding, we made a humble start and soon this expanded nationally and internationally into a very powerful collaboration, which involved other institutions in India and the US. Another example is our association with my good friend, Prof. Salim Yusuf of McMaster University in Hamilton, Canada. What started off as a small epidemiological project in India, soon expanded to involve twenty-five countries in five continents. The study produced some of the most outstanding epidemiological and other studies on diverse topics such as heart disease, diabetes, diet and nutrition and even environmental pollution and climate change, and currently involves over 200,000 participants.

It is impossible to do justice to all our collaborators in this book but in my article 'My 40-year Journey in Diabetes Research: The Power of Collaboration' (published in the journal *Perspectives in Clinical Research* in 2018), I have listed most of our collaborators in the UK, Europe, the US, Canada, Australia, Singapore and other countries. Collaborating with multiple organizations at various levels has strengthened our work and made us confident to take risks and to leap over urgent challenges. Early in life, I learnt an important lesson: you could either have a very small cake all to yourself, or you could have a piece of a really huge cake. It often turns out that even a small piece of a big cake is much bigger than the whole of the small cake. In my forty years of experience, I have learnt that while there are pros and cons for both sides, there is also value in both. On the one hand, for instance, while international collaborations can help produce high-calibre research, there is the possibility of one losing out on studies with local impact. Personal, small studies which have local relevance and impact are important, but equally important is a willingness to be collaborative and share data, experience, expertise and knowledge and become part of a much larger group, which can answer questions much bigger than small individual studies. The whole idea of medical research is to improve treatment methods and to interrogate and revise the way we think about diseases, all so that humanity at large can benefit. There is no way this can be achieved without collaboration.

I've also found that, in all my years of collaboration, any fears of being upstaged or having one's precious ideas stolen are unfounded. I have trusted people, trusted their unique strengths, and have realized how much stronger, resilient and more prepared we are together—and how this enables us to take our medical research to newer heights.

15

Achieving the Greater Good through Empowerment

There is no power for change greater than a community discovering what it cares about.

—Margaret J. Wheatley,
American writer and management consultant

When I was working as a young doctor at my father's hospital at Royapuram in the 1980s, Mother Teresa's Missionaries of Charity worked actively in the vicinity. One day, when I was finishing my work, my secretary shocked me, saying, 'Mother Teresa is here to see you, sir.' I thought it was an April Fools' joke and didn't believe her initially, but she insisted that Mother Teresa was actually waiting outside my room. I ran out and saw the diminutive figure of Mother Teresa beaming at me, her hands folded. I immediately called her into my office but she was in a hurry. 'Dr Mohan,' she said, 'I just came to thank you and your institution for your great service of looking after the health of my sisters free of cost. They are so appreciative of your work that I thought I should come in person and thank you.' I was so stunned by Mother Teresa's humility that I was speechless. Immediately, I internally strengthened my resolve to do more for such deserving people.

So one day when Rema walked up to me and said, 'Mohan, we have to do something for rural India. All our efforts in diabetes are focused in cities. Let us develop a rural model of diabetes care,' I was ecstatic to begin our work in the rural community.

Almost 72 per cent of India's population lives in rural areas, whereas 75 per cent of the doctors in India practise in urban areas. This inherent mismatch translates into India's villages being neglected and not having access to basic healthcare, leave alone specialized diabetes care. But this isn't an easy problem to solve. In many Indian villages the availability of drinking water, electricity, education and transport facilities still remains a formidable challenge. How, then, does one motivate highly qualified doctors to move to rural areas?

A few days after I had this conversation with Rema, I got a call from a well-known lawyer and philanthropist, Mr C. Ramakrishna, who hailed from a village called Chunampet in Kanchipuram district, located about 120 kilometres south of Chennai. This communication with Mr Ramakrishna was arranged by a common friend, Mr S.S. Rajsekar, who had been successfully running the National Agro Foundation in Chunampet, on a plot of land donated by Mr Ramakrishna. Over the phone, Mr Ramakrishna invited me to come down to Chunampet to discuss a project.

Mr Ramakrishna owned large tracts of land at Chunampet, which he was donating to several organizations including schools, the government, non-governmental agencies and colleges, among others. Rajsekar had spoken to him very highly of our work and so he wanted to meet me. When we met, the first question he asked me was, 'If I were to donate a plot of land to you, what would you do with it?' This needed some thinking. But I soon came up with a plan and told him that if he gave us the land, we would ensure the development of a unique rural diabetes project, which we would call the 'Chunampet Rural Diabetes Project', and added that it would be the first of its kind in India or indeed in any developing country.

As this was a rural centre, we were also committed to run the centre in charity mode. We assured him that we would find the money to construct the building and the equipment needed for the project. Mr Ramakrishna liked our idea and donated a few acres of his land to us. Even before we built a rural centre on the land, we decided we would start a mobile diabetes clinic and provide remote consultation using telemedicine. We approached the World Diabetes Foundation (WDF) in Denmark and requested their support in establishing a telemedicine unit. The WDF had been set up with the idea of supporting deserving diabetes projects in developing countries, which could help improve the lives of less affluent people. Our project was approved and, with the support of the WDF, we fabricated, from scratch, a mobile diabetes clinic, the first of its kind, fitted with all the equipment needed to screen for diabetes and its complications. The Indian Space Research Organization donated a satellite link, which was fitted on the bus. This would help us send images in real time, from the van to our base hospital in Gopalapuram in Chennai.

The project proved to be a mega success. Within a period of two years, we were able to screen a population of 50,000 people in forty-two villages in and around Chunampet. The entire adult population was screened for diabetes, and everyone with the disease was invited to undergo a further, more thorough, screening for diabetes complications. This was also the first time we were collecting rural data on diabetes and its complications in India. We then went on to build a rural centre on the plot of land donated to us. The funds for this were donated by our family and thus was born the Sai Rural Diabetes Centre, India's first rural diabetes centre.

Those below the poverty line were treated free of cost, while all others received treatment at extremely subsidized rates. This meant that the patients were able to avail of the same services offered in Chennai or other cities at a much lower cost. Plus they saved money on travel, apart from time.

Over the last fifteen years, this rural centre has become a nucleus for population-based screening and for regular follow-up care for Chunampet and several villages around it. But what's most heartening is the interest Chunampet's residents show in the centre. A local doctor joined us after undergoing training in diabetes at our Chennai centres, taking charge of the Sai Rural Diabetes Centre. This doctor, who was practising in the area, decided to dedicate his life to his people. As he was taught all the same protocols that we follow in Chennai, he was able to easily deliver a world-class diabetes centre to the villages. Thousands of villagers, who otherwise would have had no access to diabetes treatment, now were able to receive specialized care for diabetes and its complications, right at their doorstep.

This project has won international acclaim. The Discovery Channel, CNN, BBC, the French newspaper *La Monde* and a book titled *Jugaad Innovation* have all reported on the success of the Chunampet diabetes project. In an article on healthcare in India published in the *Lancet*, the Chunampet project is highlighted as a unique and novel example of providing healthcare to the rural poor: 'The Chunampet Rural Diabetes Project thus seems to be a good model for delivering preventive and therapeutic diabetes healthcare to rural areas.'

Many leaders have dreamt of self-sufficient villages. Dr A.P.J. Abdul Kalam, the former President of India, was also one of them. His dream was for India's villages to be empowered; he introduced the concept of PURA (Provision of Urban Amenities to Rural Areas), a strategy for rural development in India. He firmly believed that if the same facilities were available in rural as well as urban areas, our country would develop more rapidly, as most of India essentially lives in its villages. Moreover, this would reduce or even stop unnecessary rural-to-urban migration. The latter is responsible for the growth of urban slums where people live in squalid conditions and suffer from numerous diseases and ill health besides adding to urban poverty and witnessing an unbridled growth in the urban population. Dr Kalam visited us in Chunampet and was extremely pleased to see how it and the surrounding villages had been transformed, thanks to the collaborative efforts of philanthropists and social workers. He praised the project, which he termed a 'model for rural upliftment', and hoped it could be scaled up to other parts of India.

The Chunampet diabetes project is a shining example of how if people from different walks of life come together with a common goal of improving lives, a lot can be done. And this is one more instance of utilizing the power of collaboration to serve mankind. The Chunampet project also reaffirmed my belief in what people can achieve if they simply have the information and the right tools at their disposal.

Let me now share another satisfying experience with regard to directly empowering people. In 1996, we took up our first epidemiological study of diabetes, the Chennai Urban Population Study, which was carried out in a middle-income housing society, the Asiad Colony in Thirumangalam, and a low-income settlement in T. Nagar in Chennai. The study showed, as expected, a significantly higher prevalence of diabetes in the middle-income group (12.4 per cent) compared to the lower-income group (6.5 per cent). The results of the study were discussed with the residents of both colonies. After the awareness campaigns, the middle-income residents realized the value of increasing physical activity. They approached the government and offered to build a park with *their* own funds. After the necessary permissions were obtained, they built a beautiful park adjacent to their colony. This helped increase not just *their* physical activity but also that of people in the entire neighbourhood!

We thought this provided us a great opportunity to do some real-world research. The research question for us was: *Did building the park help reduce, or at least slow down, the rapidly escalating diabetes epidemic in their colony?* A follow-up study was conducted after ten years, which showed that in the middle-income group where the park was created, the prevalence of diabetes only marginally increased from 12.4 to 15.4 per cent (a 24 per cent increase). At the same time, in the lower-income settlement, where no intervention was done, the prevalence of diabetes increased from 6.5 per cent to 15.3 per cent (a staggering 135 per cent increase). This shows that diabetes could be prevented from manifesting in a large number of people in Asiad Colony and the neighbouring colonies due to the park.

This study was one of the first in India to introduce a real-world lifestyle intervention in the prevention of diabetes through community empowerment. And the best part was that it was achieved with no government funding whatsoever. What else do we need to prove that when people are empowered, they can use their tremendous potential for greater good?

16

Once You Make a Promise, Never Break It

Promise is a big word. It either makes something or it breaks everything.

—Anonymous

One evening, when I was studying in the sixth standard, I met one of my father's patients. My father introduced me to him, casually mentioning that I was studying at St Mary's High School on Armenian Street. The gentleman responded that his office was very close to my school. He then asked me what my hobbies were. When I mentioned that I collect stamps and coins from different countries, he replied that he, too, was a collector and had a large number of spare stamps and coins which he would be very happy to pass on to me. He then invited me to his office.

The next day, after school, I fixed an appointment with his secretary and went to meet him. I was made to wait for a long time, which of course I did not mind because I knew he was a busy man. After about an hour, he called me inside and apologized profusely, saying that he had forgotten to bring the stamps and coins with him and asked me to come back the following day. When I arrived the next day, once again, I was made to wait for an interminably long time, only to be told that he had again forgotten the items. This went on for several days, and every time I went in to see him, it was the same story. It was only after the tenth such attempt or so that I realized that the man was probably playing the fool with me and had no intention of giving me either the stamps or the coins. I was deeply hurt, not because I did not get the stamps or coins but because I had not even asked for them in the first place. It was *he* who had offered them to me. It was *he* who invited me to his office. And yet he chose to cheat me—a mere young schoolboy.

Similarly, when I was in the ninth standard, all the students were given targets by our teachers, to try and collect advertisements for the school magazine. I approached my father's friend, a businessman, asking him whether he would be willing to place an advertisement in our magazine. He readily agreed, filled out the form and gave me the material for the advertisement. It was promptly published. He had promised to make the payment as soon as a copy of the magazine reached him. I collected a few copies of the magazine and approached the gentleman with the invoice. When I met him, he gave me an appointment for a few days later. When I went again on the appointed time and date, he made an excuse and turned me away. I returned to his office in this manner no less than a dozen times over the next few months—but he would not make the payment. As a schoolboy I did not possess the inner strength or wherewithal to take him on. Eventually, as pressure from the school mounted, I ended up paying the money myself from the meagre amount I had saved from my pocket money, birthday collection and other gifts.

These two events made a lasting impression on me and I decided that I would never behave like the two gentleman. I made a vow to myself that if I ever made a promise to someone, I would keep that promise at all costs. Throughout my life I have tried to follow this principle. I cannot remember a single instance when I have failed to keep my promise and have tried on every occasion to keep my word. It is amazing how childhood impressions can last a lifetime.

My youthful experiences came to a head when my wife, Rema, and I left my father's centre and ventured out on our own. We didn't have any money but plenty of promises from our family and friends about how they would help us. When I approached my close relatives for financial assistance, they promptly turned me down. I then hoped to find help from friends. The first friend I approached was ecstatic about our plans and encouraged me to start at the earliest. And when I showed him the blueprint, he seemed to jump at it and readily promised that he would make the investments himself. He was so earnest with his promises and commitment that even a flicker of doubt did not cross my mind. But the days turned into weeks and we were given only excuses, no investments. It took me some time to realize that our friend had no intention of investing with us at all. The manner in which he had promised me was so convincing that I had refused to believe that he would go back on his word. At no point had he made me feel that he wasn't interested. It was a sad realization, that there are a lot of people in the world who will not hesitate to make promises and will go back on their word immediately afterwards, without so much as batting an eyelid.

Multiple such experiences in my life have convinced me that when we keep our word, not only do we earn the respect of people but we also make a statement about ourselves: that we are trustworthy, reliable and earnest about commitment. This, in the long run, earns the trust of friends, colleagues and of course family.

But if there are people who deceive, there are also enough people who go out of their way to help you. These good Samaritans will always be remembered gratefully and far more than those few who stir up disappointment. When we were in the UK for our training, we had very limited funding as very small amounts of foreign exchange were given by the government at the time. The little money we had soon ran out and we were practically broke. I reached out to some relatives to seek a loan, but was met with outright refusal. And then I casually met an acquaintance at a party. Seeing my plight, he offered to help with a loan and asked me to come over to his house the following day.

Memories of the disappointments I faced during my schooldays filled my brain. However, desperate as I was, I decided to pay him a visit. I was so surprised when this gentleman, who was merely a friend of a friend, gave me a cheque for a decent sum of money. He did not even mention when I should return the money to him. If we hadn't received this timely help from this kind soul, we would have had to pack our bags and return to India. Needless to say, I paid him the entire amount back in due course.

Years later, he returned to India and settled down in Chennai and came to consult me for his diabetes. I offered to make him a shareholder in our company, which he agreed to. Till his death, he remained a loyal friend and supporter of our centre. For several years after his passing, his children continued to hold his shares, which they willingly gave up years later when I offered to buy them back. It is people like him who restored my faith in humanity, and showed me the power of making and keeping a promise, and how the solidarity that it generates binds us together.

17

There Is No Substitute for Hard Work

A dream doesn't become reality through magic; it takes sweat, determination and hard work.

—Colin Powell, sixty-fifth
Secretary of State of the United States

To be successful in life, you don't need to be gifted, but you definitely have to work hard. I realized this early in my career. And since I was fond of multitasking, I learnt to work harder than most others. I had to do justice to all the tasks I wished to pursue.

I also learnt that there is no 'one' definition of success, except the one you create for yourself. People who are unsuccessful blame everyone else except themselves for their failures. People who are successful praise everyone else but themselves. Those who are conventionally unsuccessful see successful people—those with money, power or fame—and convince themselves and others that their success was due to sheer good fortune. They attribute everything to the lucky star under which they were born or to some godfather who constantly helped them along the way. I have heard people say things like, 'If I were in that person's shoes, I would also have been successful.'

It is true that it is often our circumstances that pave the way for our success. But even during such moments of serendipity, unless we seize the opportunity and then put in our full effort and focus on what we want to achieve, success may still elude us. Little else can take you closer to the success you imagine than hard work.

When I was in medical college, I didn't imagine myself only as a doctor. I saw myself as multiple people—as a doctor, a scientist, an academician and teacher, an administrator, an entrepreneur and a leader. And I still continue to chase that dream of dabbling in multiple jobs and creating the impact that transcends traditionally created boundaries. At the time of writing this book, I still see patients several days in the week and my team members and I publish at least fifty to sixty good-quality research articles a year. That's over one research paper every week. None of this is possible without utilizing every single minute of my waking day.

In the early days of my practice, I would reach the hospital at 6.45 a.m., ready to personally greet the first patient who walked in, note down their clinical history and complete a physical examination. By 7 p.m., I would have clocked in a twelve-hour workday, with short breaks for lunch and tea. Today, with many assistants and a large team to help me, I arrive at my centre by 9.30 a.m. (or even earlier when required), and work doesn't end even after the sun sets. Then, and now, I continue to put in at least a couple of hours of work after dinner to research, read or work on administrative matters. This is the schedule I follow with very little variation. While for people in other professions weekends usually mean family time, this is not true for a doctor. I have spent many holidays working, either seeing patients or conducting some academic sessions or doing research. I usually work through most festivals and national holidays. And on many Sundays I travel, giving lectures at various national and international conferences, teaching or conducting medical-education sessions. If I have the good fortune of staying at home, I devote that Sunday to reading and writing my research papers or writing books like the one you are holding in your hand.

This isn't just my life. All doctors have to be prepared to compromise on sleep and family time if the occasion demands it. There have been innumerable occasions when I have come home tired and ready to hit the bed, when an urgent phone call from the hospital about somebody being seriously ill has sent me straight back to the hospital. Multiple times I have had to excuse myself from family events to attend a critically ill patient or make a research presentation or attend a government meeting. This is the life of doctor—and I often tell my students and junior doctors that if they want to be good doctors, they have to be prepared for a life of sacrifices.

But my life is more than just seeing and treating patients. As I am a researcher, a large chunk of my day also goes into working on research articles, and I have to masterfully make time to do this. This is why I constantly work on flights. I frequently travel within India and make several trips abroad. On a single flight to New Delhi from Chennai, I can get about two and a half hours of uninterrupted time without the distractions of phone calls or other work. This means that on the trip I will get an assured five hours (two and a half hours while going and the same amount while returning) of catching up on pending reading, correcting drafts or drumming up new ideas for research.

In addition to my own research work, I often work with students on their theses. This means reading voluminous PhD theses, running longer than 200 pages, not once, but several times, in order to spot errors and improve the presentation. My own research papers, before they are finally submitted for publication, usually go through a minimum of ten to fifteen drafts.

My father once told me, 'Mohan, don't publish a paper just to get another publication. First, every paper must carry a message.

Second, ask yourself how this paper will benefit the person who has diabetes.' These guiding principles continue to ring in my ears. Hence, every time I think of writing a research paper, I pose these questions to myself before proceeding with it.

My friends ask me why I spend so much time and wind up with so many drafts of the paper. Isn't that the job of the reviewer or the editor to pick up those errors or offer suggestions? No, I tell them, I do not agree. Anything we do—seeing a patient, writing a paper, making a presentation—is like a work of art. The painting of a master. Have Leonardo da Vinci or Vincent van Gogh ever exhibited an unfinished painting? They toiled hard and always strove for perfection, which is why their names are etched in letters of gold.

It's the same with the work that doctors or researchers do. We may not be a da Vinci or a van Gogh but we take pride in everything we do. We continually strive for excellence. But, alas, excellence is like a mirage. When we think we have achieved it, the bar automatically shifts higher and one has to continue a lifelong journey in pursuit of excellence. Of course, there's always an element of luck. There have been instances where I thought my research paper was mediocre but surprisingly received glowing feedback from the reviewers. On other occasions, what I believed to be a masterly paper was ripped apart by some who thought it was a rubbish idea. The road to success in research is strewn with the corpses of papers which were meticulously slaughtered by our peers—the reviewers and editors!

On an average, three to four reviewers analyse any paper submitted to a journal. With over 1320 publications, it means that our accepted papers would have been circulated among at least 5000 reviewers! If I add all the rejections I have received, the number can be multiplied severalfold. But it's thrilling to note that several thousand reviewers have had a hand in reviewing

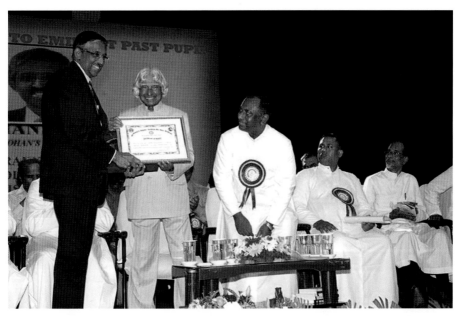

Dr Mohan being honoured as the 'Best Student Ever' of St Mary's High School, Chennai, by Dr A.P.J. Abdul Kalam, former President of India, during the 175th anniversary celebrations of the school. Father Gregory, principal of St Mary's High School, is also in the picture

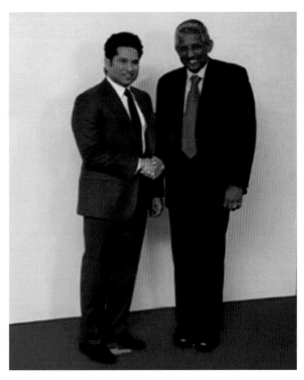

A memorable picture with Sachin Tendulkar, the cricket legend

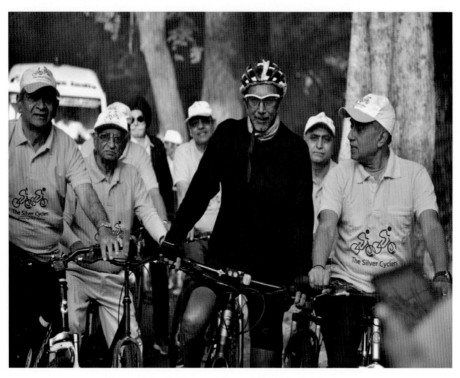

Hari Baskaran at age seventy, on his cyclothon from Chennai to Delhi

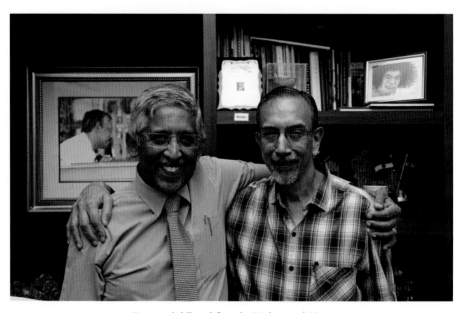

Bosom childhood friends, Mohan and Hari

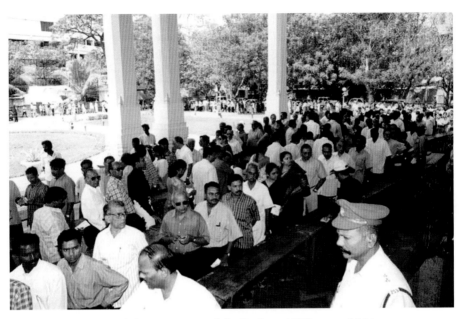

The crowds lining up to attend the 'Diabetes 2000' mega exhibition

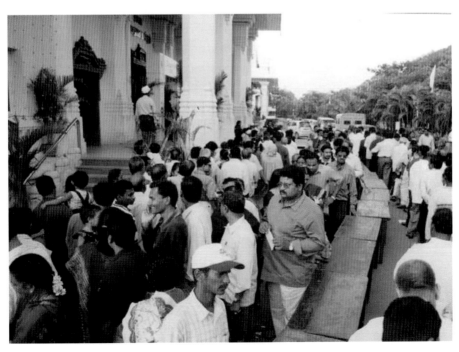

Another view of the crowd which stretched a kilometre long . . .

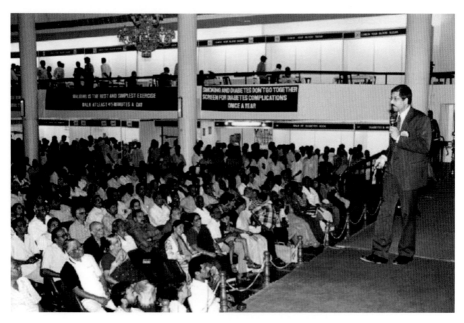

Taking diabetes to the public, as recommended by the WHO

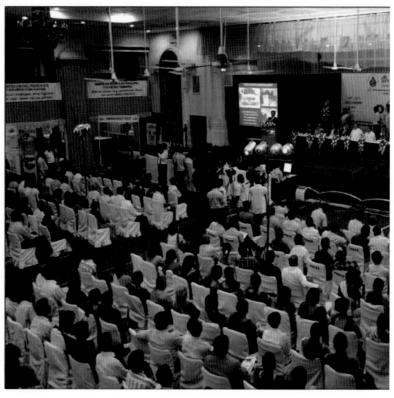

The public's eagerness to learn about diabetes was a humbling experience

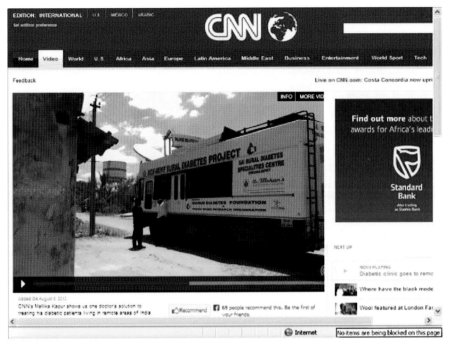

The Chunampet project covered by CNN

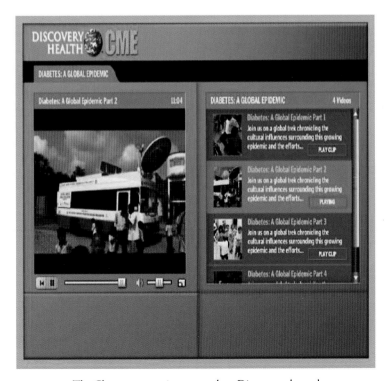

The Chunampet project covered on Discovery channel

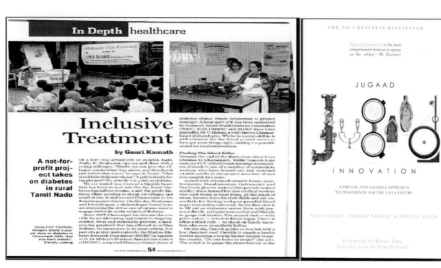

Business India on the Chunampet project

The Chunampet project highlighted in *Jugaad Innovation*

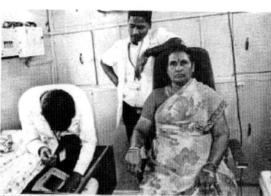

The Chunampet project covered in *Le Monde* (French newspaper)

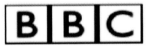

**BBC News Online
14.11.08**

India battles diabetes 'epidemic'

By Adam Mynott
BBC News, Chennai, India

Video clip here

Inside an Indian mobile diabetes clinic

Coverage of the Chunampet project by BBC News

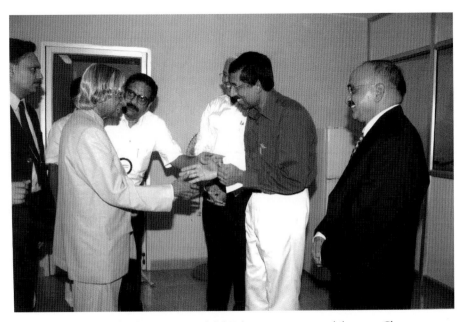

Former President of India, Dr A.P.J. Abdul Kalam, visiting our mobile van at Chunampet

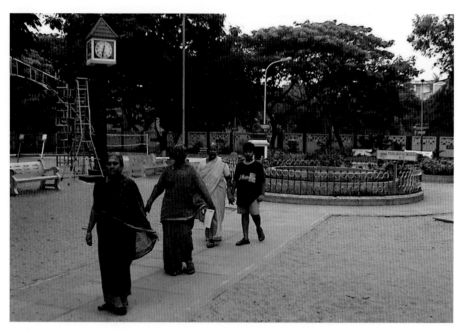

The Asiad Colony park, built by the residents of the colony—a record of sorts

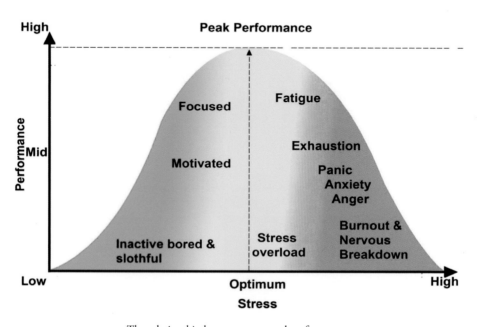

The relationship between stress and performance

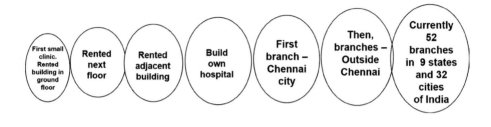

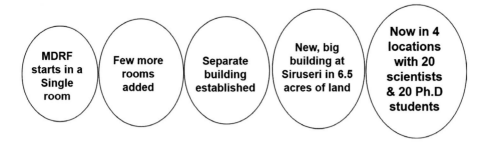

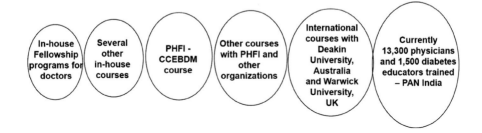

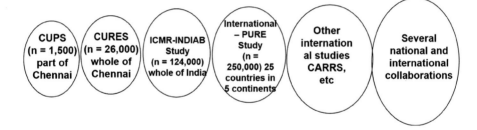

How we started small in everything we did—and how they then snowballed into mega projects

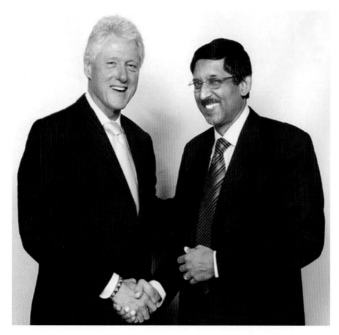

Meeting the former American President, Mr Bill Clinton, in March 2007, was an exhilarating experience

WILLIAM JEFFERSON CLINTON

April 25, 2007

Dr. V. Mohan
Number 6B
Conran Smith Road
Gopalapuram, Chennai   600086

Dear Dr. Mohan:

Thank you for the decorative plate -- it's beautiful! You were so kind to think of me, and I appreciate all the work you do to help those affected by diabetes.

All the best to you.

Sincerely,

Bill Clinton

A personal letter from Mr Bill Clinton

NUTRITION FOUNDATION OF INDIA

C. Gopalan, F.R.S.
M.D. (Madras), D.Sc. (London)
F.R.C.P. (London and Edin.)
President

Dr.V.Mohan
Dr.Mohan's Diabetes Specialities Centre
6 B Conran Smith Road,
Gopalapuram
Chennai 600086

Dear Dr.Mohan,   May 3, 2010

I am writing this to invite you to deliver the C.RAMACHANDRAN MEMORIAL LECTURE on the Annual Day of Nutrition Foundation of India, at New Delhi in the last week of November 2010.

There is mounting evidence that there has been an escalation in the incidence of diabetes in recent years, and that this is at least partly attributable to the 'nutrition transition'. You have done extensive work in this field, and I am very happy to invite you to share with us your insights on this emerging problem. Dr. Prema Ramachandran, Director of NFI, will write and give you the details of the lecture.

Your father, Dr.Viswanathan, was a good friend of mine in the days when he was working with Dr.Paul at Stanley Hospital. I am glad that you are following in the excellent tradition set by him.

With regards,

C Gopalan
C.GOPALAN

C- 13, Qutab Institutional Area, New Delhi - 110016
Tel: 26962615, 26851035 Tel/Fax: 26857814
E-mail : nutritionfoundationofindia@gmail.com, nfi@nutritionfoundationofindia.res.in
Website: www.nutritionfoundationofindia.res.in

One of my most treasured letters . . .

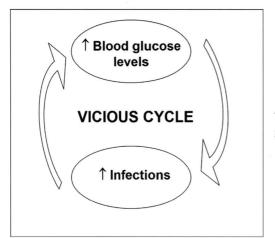

The vicious cycle between high glucose levels and infections

The functions of the conscious mind and subconscious mind

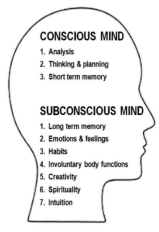

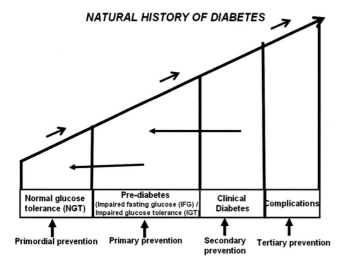

The natural history of diabetes explained

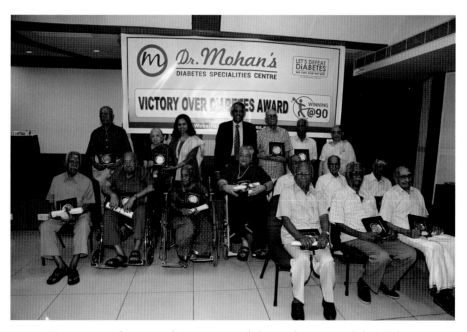

Honouring our heroes, aged ninety years and above, who conquered their diabetes

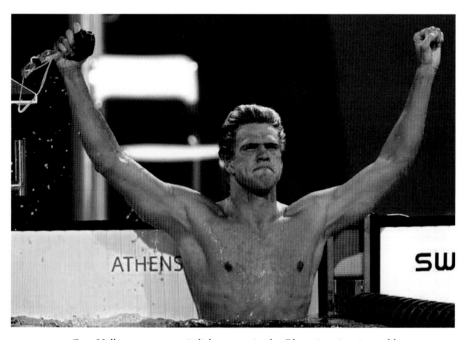

Gary Hall overcame type 1 diabetes to win the Olympic swimming gold

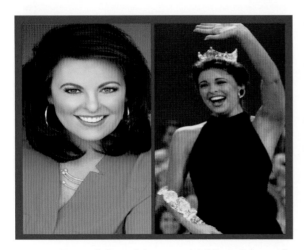
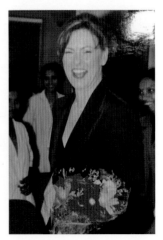

Type 1 diabetes did not stop Ms Nicole Johnson from becoming Miss America

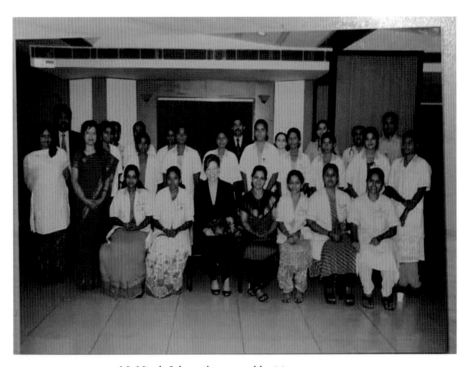

Ms Nicole Johnson's memorable visit to our centre

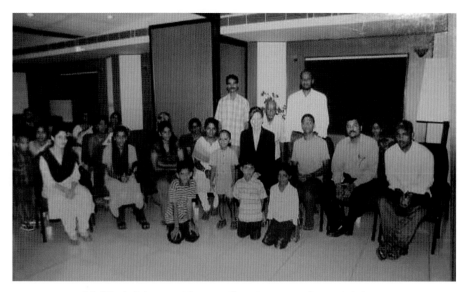

Ms Nicole Johnson with some of our tiny tots with type 1 diabetes

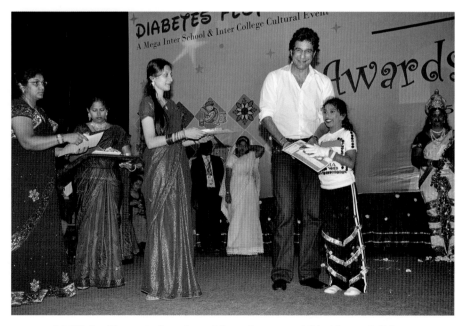

Mr Wasim Akram, the legendary cricketer, honours a child with type 1 diabetes

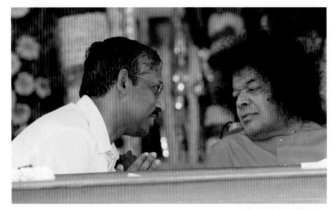

My greatest treasure—my guru, Bhagawan Sri Sathya Sai Baba

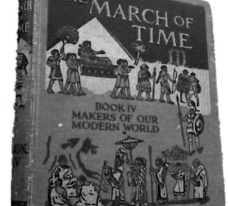

The March of Times

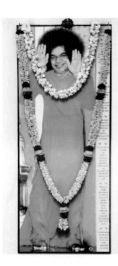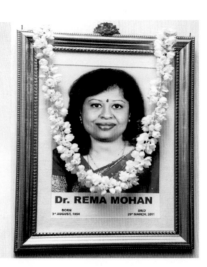

Photographs of Bhagawan Baba and my wife, Rema—the shaking-garland miracle my papers in my lifetime! This indirectly means that that many scientists from all over the world are familiar with our research. A humbling thought indeed!

Most of my doctor friends complain that they do not have the time to do research. I believe that if one has the passion and puts in hard work, it is possible to combine multiple jobs and do justice to all of them. And if there's a strong desire to gain expertise, even bestselling author Malcolm Gladwell's 10,000-hour formula to achieve excellence seems a plausible feat to me.

18

Stress and Diabetes

Stress exacerbates any problem, whether it's diabetes, heart trouble, or whatever.

—Mary Ann Mobley, American actress, television personality

A few years ago, an elderly lady walked into my room for her first diabetes consultation. It struck me as most unusual that in both hands she was holding two large 1.5-litre bottles of water, which she put down on the table with a thud. It was not a common sight and so I gently broached the subject. 'Doctor, I feel so thirsty,' she said. 'Even these two bottles of water are not sufficient for me.' When her lab tests came in, I knew the reason for her unusual thirst. Her blood sugars were above 600 mg/d l (33.3 mmol/l)! People with such high sugar levels are bound to suffer from extreme thirst, increased frequency of urination and tiredness. I requested her to immediately get admitted to the hospital. With such grossly elevated blood levels, there was a definite risk of slipping into a diabetic coma.

Once she was admitted, I started treating her with intravenous fluids and insulin injections. However, despite spending four to five days in the hospital, her blood sugars refused to come down beyond a certain level. Increasing the insulin dose and adding various anti-diabetic tablets, too, didn't help reduce the sugar levels. However, as her symptoms (thirst) had come down substantially, I discharged her at that point, advising her to continue with the insulin dosage and tablets and return after a month for her next review. When she came to see me the following month, her sugar levels had, thankfully, started coming down. Over the course of the next to two to three months, her blood sugar managed to come completely under control. Slowly, I reduced the dose of insulin and eventually withdrew it completely. Soon, the tablets were also reduced, and about a year after she had first arrived, holding the two large water bottles in her hands, her blood sugar level was completely normal, even after stopping all anti-diabetic drugs.

I was curious to know if she still had diabetes and so I did an oral glucose tolerance test, which is performed to check whether one in an early stage of diabetes. To my surprise, the test was normal and she did not have even a trace of diabetes! It was as if I was dealing with a completely different person. Here was a patient who saw me with blood glucose levels of over 600 mg/dl which insulin, tablets, a strict diet and careful hospital observation and treatment couldn't control—but the very same patient, a year later, had thrown the disease out of her body!

This was the first time I was witnessing such a dramatic reversal of diabetes. It was so baffling that I simply and stolidly asked for an explanation. Some people are intuitive and deeply aware of what's wrong with them, as was she. 'Doctor, I haven't told you the truth,' she began, and proceeded to tell me of her deep mental agony. Her husband was having an extramarital affair, and the knowledge of this had stirred a deep anguish inside her, and this was perhaps what had precipitated the diabetes in her. She had forgotten how to look after herself and both her diet and sleep schedule had been jeopardized. But something still puzzled me. 'How has your diabetes disappeared now?' I asked. 'The affair ended,' she answered coyly, with a sheepish smile. 'The woman was transferred to another city and eventually my husband lost interest in her.' I haven't forgotten this incident because it opened my eyes to the close relationship between stress and diabetes.

It's now evident that extreme stress derails the metabolic balance within our system and the biochemistry goes completely haywire. Many stress hormones in our body like cortisol, adrenaline (epinephrine) and noradrenaline (norepinephrine) get released in excessive quantities during severe stress. These stress hormones have an anti-insulin effect and oppose the action of insulin such that even if one's body is producing insulin, it is rendered ineffective by these counter-regulatory hormones. When this stress passes, the effect of counter-regulatory hormones decreases, the insulin once again becomes effective and the body is cured of diabetes.

Doctors often make the mistake of not inquiring if the patient is under unnecessary or unusual stress while diagnosing them. It's probably also because we don't understand stress ourselves. When we see increasing sugar levels in our patients, we tend to blindly increase the dose of anti-diabetic medications without attempting to find the root cause and treating it. In many cases of stress-induced diabetes, the correct treatment is to introduce 'stress control' measures, including deep-breathing exercises, as I learnt myself.

A few years ago, a friend gifted me a small device, which was like a coin that could be held between one's fingers for a few seconds. Once the pressure of the finger was released, the colour on the disc had to be observed. If it was green, it meant one was completely relaxed. And if one was stressed, the colour progressively changed to yellow, orange and then red. And if one was extremely stressed, the colour would turn black. When I first received this, I showed it to Rema, who wouldn't believe it would work. We tested it on ourselves on a relaxed Sunday evening and the green colour indicated that we were perfectly calm and happy. Both Rema and I were sceptical. 'I don't believe this,' she said. 'I think it's crap.'

The next day, I took the device to my clinic and decided to test it there. It can be quite stressful to reach the clinic and see a long queue of patients waiting outside—in short, it was the perfect moment to check the efficacy of the device. As expected, I found that the colour flashing was black. Rema was surprised to see that such a simple device could measure one's stress and we both decided to unravel the science behind it. We learnt that it worked through bioimpedance, which is the measure of how well the body impedes electric current flow. When one is stressed, minute quantities of sweat break out in the body, which the body (the fingers in this case) is able to pick up on. Now I knew that the device could capture if a person was stressed or not, but I wanted to see if the reverse was also possible. I went inside my office and started my breathing exercises. After about five to ten minutes of deep breathing and relaxation, I took out the device and tested it again and found that the colour had already turned yellow.

Since then, I have carried out a few more experiments at various times of the day and have found that breathing exercises or pranayama can bring down stress levels drastically. Pranayama, today, is part of my daily routine. Within minutes of breathing consciously and deeply, I find that my body is completely relaxed, ready to take on the day's stresses without a pang of anxiety or frustration. Naturally, I recommend breathing exercises to all my patients, to not only reduce blood pressure, heart rate and blood sugar levels, but to simply be able to work and live well. And my belief is reaffirmed every time I see patients whose diabetes has been under control for many years until a stressful situation that affected the patient's social life, sleep schedule and general state of well-being wrecked it.

But not all stress is bad. The right amount of stress has been proven to improve performance among many individuals of varying professions.

It's when stress increases and fatigue and exhaustion set in that both health and performance drop. Burnout, then, is not far away. Success, I now know, lies in tiptoeing over harmful stressors and mastering life and work with just the right amount of stress.

19

Learning to Laugh

Laugh at yourself first, before anyone else can.

—Elsa Maxwell, American columnist,
songwriter and professional hostess

Doctors are surrounded by misery and suffering. If most day-to-day lives are a struggle to stave off stress or the burden of existence, a doctor is precariously walking the tightrope of death and life. Work swallows my days and weeks and, before I know it, I find that months have elapsed since I last laughed heartily. But one of my life's key learnings is to learn to laugh. And to laugh at myself—particularly when I have embarrassed myself. And during such moments, I think about how important it is to not take yourself or life too seriously.

When I was working at the Hammersmith Hospital and the Royal Postgraduate Medical School, London, in 1984–85, I was a frequent visitor to the library. And since I took notes in longhand then (and even now), I used to carry reams of paper. At that time, if you needed to make photocopies of any articles that you were referencing, you had to mark the pages that had to be photocopied and the librarian would keep them ready for you later that day or the following day. On one such occasion, I had picked up several issues of different journals and taken down copious notes. I carried the sheaf of papers to the librarian to receive photocopies, put them down and gave her the journals to be photocopied. But just as I was stepping out of the library, a loud siren went off and everyone in the library turned to see what had happened. Apparently, *I* had set off the alarm. I stood there, petrified, not understanding what was happening. The librarian walked up to me and asked me if I had taken any issue of the journal by mistake. I replied that I had not. She then looked at my sheets and, lo and behold, at the bottom of the papers, was a brand-new journal issue. It was lying on the librarian's desk and had somehow got mixed up with my papers. The alarm went off because the library had magnetized its books and journals, and if anybody left the premise with an unchecked journal that was not demagnetized, the alarm would go off.

I had inadvertently picked up the journal, but to people using the library, it might have appeared like I was trying to steal it! However, the librarian was quite sweet and gave me the benefit of the doubt, thus saving the day for me. Thirty years have passed since this incident but I still haven't forgotten it. This is what embarrassing moments do—they leave you wishing you were dead in the moment; but then they remind you of how alive and full of life you were and make you chuckle years after the incident occurred. This episode taught me to always check my belongings and ensure I haven't mistakenly taken something that doesn't belong to me.

Similarly, I was once at an international conference which was being held at a huge convention centre. And although the place had a beautiful interior, its signages left much to be desired. It was particularly difficult to find (and identify) the restrooms. I had just given a talk and had walked out of one of the halls. Without noticing the signs properly, I walked straight into the ladies' restroom. I can never forget the look on the faces of the women inside. There was horror, shock, anger, surprise and amusement. I left hastily but just as I came out, some more women and men noticed me, which added to my embarrassment. Ever since then, I always double-check the signage on a restroom.

As a child, too, I often embarrassed myself. When I was ten years old, my father took me to Stanley Medical College for their Annual Day celebrations and sports events. One of their events, a 50-metre race, was meant for the teachers' children. Off I went to take part in the race, but to my utter embarrassment I found that most of the children, except for me, were tiny tots, aged four to six. And here I was, a towering ten-year-old—almost double their size. I offered to opt out of the race but the organizers would not hear of it. In retrospect, this was one of the most unfair races that I have ever participated in. When the bell went off, I was charging ahead. And when I was at the finish line, the unfortunate young children were only at the halfway mark. I was so embarrassed that I didn't want to go up to receive my prize. But I was made to go. Standing on the victory podium with children half my size is one of the most embarrassing moments that I can recall from my childhood.

As a doctor, now, I experience fewer and fewer such embarrassing moments. I am a patient doctor, and even if patients ask me the same question a hundred times, I calmly explain it to them, over and over again. I rarely lose my temper with a patient. But sometimes, there are patients who can drive you up the wall with their nagging. I had tolerated one such elderly lady for about twenty years. Every time she came to my room, I was certain that she would ask me the same question on a loop for the next half an hour. One day, out of sheer desperation, I decided to refer her to a diabetologist colleague. I told her that she needed a second opinion and thus I was referring her to a someone else. I wrote a carefully worded letter explaining her history and sent her off to my colleague. I was relieved that I had finally got rid of this patient. But three days later she returned to my clinic, clutching a letter in her palm.

The letter read, 'Dear Dr Mohan, I'm referring the patient back to you for a third opinion. I think you're better suited and qualified to treat her than me.' The diabetologist had seen through my bluff. I could barely contain my laughter, but the amusement was soured by a depressing reality: that it's just not possible to get rid of some problems in life. We just have to grin and bear it.

But if a few patients can drive me up the wall, I am sure I can have the same effect on patients too. Once I had insensitively told a patient's attendant, 'Madam, please ensure that your husband follows his diet and exercises regularly.' She gave me an icy look and answered, 'He is my father.'

History repeated itself years later when I took my daughter, Anjana, to a five-star hotel. She had won a prestigious prize and we wanted to celebrate. The waiter, obviously trying to be friendly, asked us, 'What's the occasion? Is it your wedding anniversary?' And this time it was my daughter's turn to give the waiter a if-looks-could-kill-you-would-be-dead-by-now kind of stare and tell him, 'He happens to be my father.' We all live to learn!

20

Start Small and Then Take Bigger Steps: The Snowball Effect

Life is like a snowball. The important thing is finding wet snow and a really long hill.

—Warren Buffett, American investor,
business tycoon, philanthropist

When I look back on the forty years I have been in the medical profession, I am convinced of one rule which worked well for me and which I think will work for you as well. If you want to achieve something substantial in life, it is always better to start small. You may have a vision of a much larger picture even in the beginning, but it is still preferable to start small. This strategy is also, in some ways, a shield against miserable, brutal failure. There is no guarantee of success and, often, when we are deeply invested in something, it's difficult to extricate ourselves from the certainty of failure and from the mess it leaves behind. There's a reason why starting small is considered the first step towards greatness.

The lives of many artists and renowned personalities confirm this mantra: Vincent van Gogh had said: 'Great things are not done by impulse, but by a series of small things brought together.' An old Chinese proverb goes: 'It is better to take many small steps in the right direction than to make a great leap forward, only to stumble backward.' And we all know the famous Chinese philosopher Lao Tzu, who said, 'The journey of a thousand miles begins with one step.'

I took my first step as an entrepreneur when Rema and I started our small clinic in 1991. We rented a building and occupied one floor. When this succeeded, we rented the next floor and, soon, an adjacent building. From there, the next step was to buy a piece of land and build our hospital. Finally, we started our expansion programme and opened multiple branches of our centre. The first one in another part of Chennai, the next in another city, Hyderabad, and, finally, we established branches in many other cities and states in India. If we now trace the growth of our institutions, it all started with the first small clinic. This then snowballed into a large chain of diabetes centres all over the country.

In his well-known book *Influence: The Psychology of Persuasion*, Robert B. Cialdini explains, 'Start by taking the smallest possible action towards your goal and then leverage that commitment to motivate yourself to do more.' Cialdini's book elaborates on the social psychology research which points to the fact that even a small action creates commitment in us towards that action and this then drives us to continue to develop that idea. We tiptoe around an idea first and then, slowly, gradually, do we dip our feet, and it's only after finding firm grounding that we can proceed, even if that requires first wading through muddy waters.

Regardless of the areas I worked in medical practice—research or education—I have experienced a similar snowball effect. The Madras Diabetes Research Foundation started in one room of our hospital with one staff member. It then grew rapidly and soon had its own building. Today, it is spread over four locations in Chennai, with over twenty scientists and twenty PhD students at any given time. However, this growth occurred over a period of years and followed a particular pattern, building on the strengths of our earlier successes and what had been achieved.

In education and capacity-building as well, through the Dr Mohan's Diabetes Education Academy, we first started our own in-house training programmes for doctors and later expanded this through our collaborations with the Public Health Foundation of India. We established a certification course in evidence-based diabetes management (CCEBDM), which led to other courses with the PHFI, in addition to courses for diabetes educators, nurses and paramedical professionals, with assistance from different organizations and universities.

In specific research areas, too, we started small. Take epidemiology, for instance. We started with a small epidemiological research project, the Chennai Urban Population Study (or CUPS), with a small sample size of around 1500 participants. This made way for a study of the whole of Chennai—the Chennai Urban Rural Epidemiology Study (or CURES), with a sample size of 26,000. We didn't stop there. On my daughter Anjana's insistence, we aimed higher and conducted an epidemiological study of diabetes in the whole of India: the Indian Council of Medical Research–INdia DIABetes (or ICMR–INDIAB) study, with a sample size of 1,24,000 participants, which was truly representative of India's 1.34 billion people.

It is now my conviction that when we start small, we have a steeper learning curve, during which we can find out our strengths and weaknesses. We also gradually develop confidence in doing things smarter and better. Our teams also gain confidence that they can take on bigger and bigger challenges, grow and achieve mind-boggling success.

Mark Twain sums up this concept of starting small and then snowballing beautifully:

> Evolution is a blind giant who rolls a snowball down a hill. The ball is made of flakes—circumstances. They contribute to the mass without knowing it. They adhere without intention, and without foreseeing what is to result. When they see the result they marvel at the monster ball and wonder how the contriving of it came to be originally thought out and planned. Whereas there was no such planning, there was only one law: the ball once started, all the circumstances that happened to lie in its path would help to build it, in spite of themselves.

But even as we start small and gradually try to widen our horizons, there are qualities we must remember from the time we were still finding our feet. One such quality is humility, and in fact the world's greatest people adhere to this simple principle. In 2007, I received an invitation to attend a prestigious diabetes meeting to be held in New York. Very soon, I found out that the former US President Bill Clinton would be the chief guest addressing the meeting and would also be personally interacting with the few select doctors who were also invited to participate. I was lucky to have been invited and, on the day, some thirty-odd doctors were introduced to Mr Clinton.

On the day, I was carrying a present for Mr Clinton but his security stopped me from taking it to him, or directly handing it over, till it had been checked. But they promised me that it would be delivered to him. I met Mr Clinton without the gift and, while we were chatting, he got a phone call on his mobile phone. It turned out that the former US President George Bush Sr was on the line. Mr Clinton excused himself, took the call and returned, apologetic, for keeping me waiting. I told him about the gift and thanked him for the work his foundation was doing for the tsunami victims.

Mr Clinton, in turn, was all praise for the Tamil Nadu government for their tsunami relief operations. After the introductions, Mr Clinton gave a dazzling opening address, replete with statistics and technical know-how—all without a cue card in his hand. One could not help but admire the charisma and knowledge of the man.

A few days after the meeting, I was surprised to receive a personal letter from Mr Clinton, thanking me for the gift. Since then, I have written to Mr Clinton a couple of times and have always received a reply.

Every time I think about my meeting with him, I am reminded of the traits that lead to greatness: from the courtesy he showed me by apologizing for making me wait to remembering to thank me for a gift—these are all traits that help people rise to greatness. Like everyone else, Bill Clinton, too, started small before he rose to become the US President. But he didn't forget where he came from—and his humility shone through his personality.

21

Team Building

Coming together is a beginning. Keeping together is progress. Working together is success.

—Henry Ford, American industrialist
and founder of the Ford Motor Company

How is it that large, dispersed teams in top-of-the-rung medical institutions manage a flurry of activity smoothly? How do they coordinate patient care, the expansion of the clinics, research, education and charity, all at the same time? The secret to building any institution is the camaraderie or teamwork that keeps them fuelled. The main reason why we have been able to build highly cohesive teams is because of an ethos of trust and empowerment. When Rema and I started our own institution in 1991, we had a grand total of twenty staff members, which included four doctors. The first physician diabetologist who joined me was my former student Dr N.G. Sastry, who had completed his training in diabetology at my father's institution when I was there. Dr Sastry's course completion coincided with the launch of our centre. Hence, when I requested Dr Sastry to join our centre, he readily agreed.

Over the next decade, Dr Sastry became the backbone of the diabetology services at our centre in Chennai. By this time, the institution had grown and we could sense that Dr Sastry was looking for something bigger. We asked him whether he would like to relocate to his home state, Andhra Pradesh (later divided into Telangana and Andhra Pradesh), and, if yes, we could set up a branch in Hyderabad. Sastry readily agreed to this proposal. For us, it meant instating a branch in an adjacent state, while for Sastry it meant having the independence to work as the head of our branch in his home state. It was a mutually beneficial project.

Dr Sastry quickly established himself in Hyderabad and now has a huge following of dedicated patients, some of whom even travel from Chennai and other cities in India to Hyderabad to consult him. Very soon, we were able to build our team with doctors of different levels of seniority and mentoring experience. This helped us to expand into new geographies. In each of the branches we started, the doctor who took charge of that branch would soon establish himself or herself as the leading consultant in that area. This experiment proved to be so successful that eventually we were able to attract private equity funding and grow at a much faster pace.

But the genesis of this culture of support and appreciation and team building was Rema. She walked the tightrope of being both a strict boss and a loving friend with such ease that people began to consider her family. Regardless of people's positions in the organization, Rema made everyone feel valued. A team member and ophthalmologist, Dr Rajalakshmi, remembers that despite Rema being the 'Chief', as some called her, when important department decisions had to be taken, she discussed the matter with the entire team and valued their opinions. 'Even a small achievement by the team used to be greatly recognized and appreciated,' Dr Rajalakshmi says.

This is the reason why many staff members felt compelled to stay with us despite the attraction of a higher salary elsewhere. And in turn Rema and I would be extremely grateful for the committed staff member who was willing to go the extra mile.

Lately, however, I have also uncovered a truth about team management that is often left unspoken: what is important is how you make your team members feel. The night Rema passed away, thousands of people turned up to pay their respects. Finally, at 10.30 in the night, exhausted after the cremation, I was about to close the front door and finally retire, when another visitor arrived. I was surprised to see that he was a staff member who had worked with us several years ago. He apologized for being late and said he was out of town. The second he heard the news, he said, he skipped his dinner and rushed to our house. He asked if he could sit for a few minutes in front of Rema's picture; I agreed. He sat down in meditation in front of the picture, and to me it felt like a long time passed before he even stirred. Finally, when he got up, he said two words: 'Thank you.' And left. The incident had a profound impact on me. He was a former staff member at our centre, and while I hadn't interacted with him much, Rema had clearly connected with him deeply—just as she did with everyone. It was obvious that he, too, valued her deeply and was thus compelled to pay his respects even at that late hour. At that moment, I realized how many lives the institution—and Rema—had touched and how she continued to inspire people towards achieving greatness.

But as the organization has grown, so have the challenges of keeping up with this kind of personal interaction with our staff. Today, we are located in thirty-two different cities in India, and I often worry about being able to connect with everyone. It's a key reason why every year, when I address our staff on founder's day, I don't miss the opportunity to talk about teamwork. I repeatedly emphasize to people that it is the team which is important. And if the team clicks, we win. If the team doesn't, we lose. Some doctors might be competent medically, but if they're not team players, they will constantly find fault with others and demoralize them, or chase personal glory, leading to the splintering of the team. We have seen higher attrition rates in such teams. And eventually, the branch begins to suffer and the number of visiting patients begins to go down as well.

It's not just about the doctor and the patient. It is also about the telephone operator answering calls, the front-office person who receives the patient and the dietician, technician or nurse who makes the patient feel comfortable. Each person is as important as the doctor. In some branches we have doctors who are excellent team players, who give importance and acknowledge the value addition of their team, and this helps the branch flourish.

Today, there are quite a few things we have done which have helped earn the trust and commitment of our staff. After my daughter, Dr Anjana, took over as a managing director of the centre in 2016, she introduced many new engagement initiatives for the staff. Her inspiration has been her mother, who was deeply respected and adored each and every person of the team. And like her mother, Anjana has continued to build a culture and atmosphere of communication and appreciation. A simple annual cultural celebration, for example, where the institution is divided into teams, we've found, boosts team spirit like little else. And the focus here isn't merely the doctors or those in the higher echelons of management but also the bottom rung: indeed each and every person who contributes to the organization. As teams indulge in activities, captains and vice captains ensure there's abundant participation. As a result, hidden talents are discovered, a sense of unity is fostered and the feeling of camaraderie and family is reinforced. It is teamwork at its best.

22

Combining Entrepreneurship with Ethics and Empathy

The secret of the care of the patient is in caring for the patient.

—Dr Francis Peabody, American physician known
for his research on poliomyelitis and typhoid

The traditional picture of a doctor from a few decades ago is of a jovial, often pot-bellied, middle-aged physician who is a family friend of the patient. He listens carefully to the patient's history and symptoms and then prescribes one among six or seven concoctions, usually of different colours, which the compounder dispenses. Since then, medicine has rapidly advanced, and from being an art form of sorts, it slowly evolved to become a science. And today, it has turned into a business.

In the good old days, an ECG or X-ray were seldom available, so a physician would have to make an on-the-spot diagnosis. They would take down a detailed history of the patient, feel their pulse, the blood pressure, and a detailed clinical examination would follow. Finally, a diagnosis would be made and the treatment prescribed.

As modern equipment came into medical practice, diagnosis has become sharper and more accurate. This, unfortunately, has led to a decline in the clinical acumen of doctors. Today's doctors hardly feel the need to use the stethoscope or their medical-school-acquired clinical skills and are heavily dependent on laboratory investigations and sophisticated equipment.

To be fair, there is nothing right—or wrong—with this. From a small practice, the doctor's clinic has evolved into a nursing home, a small hospital and, finally, into a multi-speciality, state-of-the-art hospital with modern facilities—a five-star hotel for the sick. From a solitary doctor, or one with at best a compounder to assist him/her, hospitals now have CEOs, multiple managers, administrators and other technical staff members.

All this of course means that the costs of setting up these institutions have ramped up prices for individuals on both sides of the table. But there are different types of doctors. Some are content just doing their clinical work, working in one of these major hospitals. And as their entire time is spent in clinical work, they do not have the time, inclination or the ability to look into matters of administration. But there are others, who, apart from being highly skilled as doctors, are also entrepreneurs who would like to run their own hospitals. Sometimes, the business takes precedence over healing as the doctor devotes his or her entire energy into building and running the hospital, managing the doctors, the paramedics and other operational duties

Early in my career, I had to make a choice. Would I be just another entrepreneur, or an entrepreneur who also heals and prioritizes people over business? A good way of knowing what you want to do is to ask yourself what you would do if you made no money out of what you are pursuing. And when I asked myself this question, the answer came through loud and clear: medicine. I decided that at no stage in my life would I give up my medical practice, as that was the very purpose of my life and the reason I entered this noble profession. But along with practising medicine, I had a second resolution: to continue to do research and publish good-quality research papers. This meant that I already had two jobs: one as a doctor seeing patients and the other as a researcher. I took up a third job, too: I became a teacher to train hundreds of doctors and other medical personnel to do what I could never hope to achieve by myself: improve the lives of millions of diabetics. This therefore became the third aspect of my personality. Fourthly, I trained myself to become an entrepreneur to run my own institutions and establish centres in different parts of the country. Finally, I also nursed the deep and intense spiritual craving to help those who couldn't afford treatment. This became my fifth job—to run free charitable clinics in both urban and rural areas. I must admit that doing five different things at the same time is physically and mentally exhausting. Never would I compromise on my medical ethics or the time spent to train and mentor others. After four decades of performing four to five different roles, I can confidently say that there's no need to restrict yourself to one job; instead, dabble in multiple avenues, provided you have the passion and energy to do each job well.

Many hospitals today are driven like a business and not as a service to people. Institutions, unless they are government-run or charitable, need money to grow, and for such institutions, the only inflow of money is what they earn by treating patients.

But this is also where the ethos of the company, the ethical principles on which the hospital is founded, comes into play. They could face a lot of temptations to prescribe unnecessary treatments to do investigations and, in some unfortunate cases, even commit blatant fraud or cause harm to the patients. Empathy and trust must come first in healthcare but, unfortunately, it's in rare supply.

We started small, as a stand-alone clinic in 1991 and then started growing slowly but steadily. We borrowed money from the bank and promptly repaid all loans. And when we reached a certain critical size, it was clear to us that we had to explore other avenues of investment. In 2017, we received our first round of private equity investment. At this point, the pressure to perform can be very high. This is also where the ethics of many companies crumble and their deepest values are put to the test.

But even as we've been trying to accentuate our incomes, it's not at the cost of ethics or doing anything that pricks the conscience. Each and every doctor who works with me knows that he or she has the total freedom to deny an unethical order, regardless of who it comes from.

In 2018, a patient from Malaysia came to see me. He had heard about insulin pumps—a small, pager-sized device with an insulin syringe inside—and how useful they were for the treatment of diabetes. These insulin pumps are battery-operated, and the dosage of insulin that is to be delivered can be measured out by adjusting the knobs on the pump. One can, for example, give more insulin in the daytime, less at night and also give a variable amount of insulin after each meal, depending on what the patient has eaten. The insulin pump, therefore, is a useful tool that helps control diabetes better and prevents unnecessary swings in blood sugar levels and, most importantly, prevents low-sugar reactions in the body.

The problem is that this device is meant for patients with type 1 (insulin-dependent) diabetes, or those with type 2 diabetes, who are in the late stages and behave clinically like type 1 patients requiring multiple doses of insulin. This patient had an early stage of type 2 diabetes. He had been prescribed small doses of tablets, and his diabetes was under excellent control. Hence, not only did he not need an insulin pump, he did not even need insulin. The man, however, was insistent that I put him on a pump.

There was no way I could concede to his demand. To begin with, I would not know how much insulin to give him and, second, since his sugars were under control, I wasn't sure if the insulin would work as well as his tablets already were. Finally, the insulin might push him into dangerously low levels of blood sugar which could even be life-threatening. I told him that there was no question of my prescribing an insulin pump for him.

The patient was furious. It turned out that he had arrived all the way from Malaysia because a friend of his had been treated at our centre and was prescribed the insulin pump. I checked his friend's notes and found that he suffered from typical type 1 insulin-dependent diabetes. That was why the pump was prescribed to him.

The cost of an insulin pump is around $3500. I could have easily sold him the pump and pocketed the money, but that would have been not only unethical but also unscientific. It was only after several rounds of discussion that I managed to convince the patient that he did not need the pump. I assured him that if his diabetes deteriorated in the future, I would be the first to initiate the pump for him. I am confident that no one at my institution would have prescribed a pump to this patient because we deeply value ethics at our organization. And along with ethics, comes a willingness to be charitable.

When we first started our institution in 1991, we also started treating some of our needy patients free of cost. It's because we felt that we should have an instinct for charity built into the ethos of our organization. While for other medical conditions, charitable treatment is one-time and final, the case of diabetes is different. Diabetes is a lifelong condition, and once we take on free treatment, it means that we must treat the patient for life. And as the years pass, the treatment gets more complicated. Initially, we would prescribe inexpensive drugs like Metformin, but when the patient came by for subsequent visits, a second drug would also be needed to get the diabetes under control. And afterwards, quite often, a third or a fourth drug would become necessary and, later, even insulin injections. The cost of the treatment would therefore shoot up astronomically. This makes it a formidable challenge to run a free clinic—where not only do the investigations have to be done for free, the consultation fees also have to be waived and the medicines handed over gratis.

While we have been fortunate enough to have had some donations flow in, most of the time, it's our own personal funding or a part of the hospital income which is utilized for providing charitable services either in our own hospital or in the charitable clinics we have set up across Chennai in conjunction with various charitable and spiritual organizations.

Since I also do clinical research, this is another opportunity where I try to be ethical and charitable. For instance, I was initially working on a condition termed 'fibrocalculous pancreatic diabetes', in which diabetes is caused due to the stones that form inside the pancreatic duct. Patients with this form of diabetes experience recurrent abdominal pain. They're usually thin and emaciated and malnourished. Most often, they are poor. As I was working for a PhD and, later, for a Doctor of Science degree, on this form of diabetes, I had a large number of patients suffering from this condition. It was because of these patients that I was able to learn so much about a rare form of diabetes. In turn, I offered them free treatment for life.

One such patient happened to meet a colleague of mine who was a surgeon. He had to undergo surgery and, once it was done, the patient paid the full fees. The surgeon then called me to boast about how the patient had paid the entire amount to him, where, on the other hand, the patient was getting free treatment from me. 'Mohan, he has fooled you.' 'Doc,' I answered, 'I think you got it wrong. The patient did not ask me for free treatment. He comes from a relatively poor background, and yet he participated in my studies and offered me his time. The least I could do was offer him free treatment.' The experience strengthened my resolve to not just provide more charitable services but also create a fund to help more poor and deserving patients. This led to the setting up of our charitable trust called the Diabetes International Research Education and Charitable Trust (DIRECT), which provides lifelong free treatment, including medicines, for thousands of poor patients.

We also extended our service to the autorickshaw drivers in Chennai. Many of them had very high blood sugar and blood pressure levels and their health condition was dangerous, not only for them, but also for the passengers who used their services. So we took up a programme along with the Sri Sathya Sai Seva Organization, where, through a series of camps, we screened over 12,000 autorickshaw drivers in Chennai and offered all those with diabetes free treatment for life.

My experiences teach me that it is through charitable work that we learn more about ourselves—our values, motivation, what drives us and of course our ethics. A charitable sensibility, ethics and the right way of doing business must seep into the fabric of any institution. Indeed, they should become its very foundation.

23

Applying 'Placebo' and
Spiritual Methods in Medical Care

The emotion that can break your heart is sometimes the very one that heals it.

—Nicholas Sparks, *At First Sight*

Many people are now familiar with what is called the 'placebo effect', but it has never failed to amaze me. For those unfamiliar with this term, let me explain what it means: when we do a randomized clinical trial (RCT) to test a new drug, usually as a comparator to the drug which is being tested, an identical-looking placebo (a control pill that does not contain the medication) is also given. When the trial is completed, undoubtedly, the medicine which is being tested would show expected effects. But what is most surprising is that the 'control arm' where individuals received the 'placebo' treatment also shows some response.

Let us say we are testing a new drug for diabetes. In Arm A, where the real pill was given, if the blood glucose reduction was 100 mg/dl, we might find that in Arm B, where the placebo pill is given, there is a 30 mg/dl reduction in blood glucose. Then the actual blood glucose reduction due to the drug is 100 minus 30, or 70 mg/dl. We term this the 'placebo subtracted effect' of the drug. Why did the placebo arm show an improvement in the first place? We do not understand this fully but it could be due to a number of mechanisms.

First, since patients receive better care as they are in a trial, it could result in some improvement in their parameters such as blood glucose levels. It could also be because the patient *believes* that he or she is getting a better drug. When the patient believes this, it could induce a blood-glucose-lowering response because the mind believes that it is receiving a treatment which will lead to an improvement. It is this 'placebo effect' which leads to improvements and even miraculous cures by faith healers. When people go to these people with the confidence that they will be cured, often a mere touch or a word spoken by them is enough to 'cure' a disease. As the placebo effect is innocuous and does not have any side effects, it can be utilized quite fruitfully. One of the ways to do this would be by using positive affirmation, autosuggestion or the power of positive thinking in healing.

Five years ago, I was reviewing the records of a patient who had been coming fairly regularly to see me. I found that her control of diabetes had always been suboptimal. A glycated haemoglobin (A1c) (an index measuring three months' control of diabetes) value of less than 7 per cent is considered an acceptable level of control for people with diabetes. This lady's A1c was always in the range of 8.5 to 10 per cent, indicating poor control of diabetes. After discussing the various treatment options with her and giving her a pep talk to achieve better diabetes control, I wrote in her case sheet: *Next time, your HbA1c will be below 7 per cent.* I got her to sign under this statement, an undertaking of sorts, and I also signed it. Three months later, she came back for her next check-up and, lo and behold, her

HbA1c was 6.8 per cent, i.e. below the 7 per cent target that I had written she would achieve! This was the first time ever that she had achieved this target. How did this happen? It is possible that since she signed the statement, she became more careful with her diet. It's also possible that she exercised more or took her medicines regularly. For eight years, she had been coming to our centre and I had tried various permutations and combinations of medications to bring her A1c down. Nothing had worked. But the simple act of writing in her case sheet that the A1c *would* come below 7 per cent worked wonders—and she achieved the target.

Another powerful tool we have successfully employed in the clinic is to use a colour code. Without the patient's knowledge, we would put a small coloured sticker on the top of the case notes. If the sticker was green it meant that the patient's A1c was below 7 per cent and therefore no change was needed. If the sticker was yellow, it meant the A1c was between 7 and 8.5, which needed some attention from our team. Finally, if it was above 8.5 per cent, we put a red sticker to indicate poor control. This was meant to be a secret code for quick identification in our busy clinic, to immediately note which patients needed more of our attention and time, in terms of lifestyle modification, counselling or change of medications. However, some curious patients noticed the stickers and were eager to know what the colours meant. We had to therefore explain it to them. One patient who had a red sticker told me, quite emphatically, that next time we would have to change her sticker colour to a green one. Three months later, when the patient came back for review, her A1c was 6.6 per cent, and indeed we had to change it to a green sticker. In many patients with diabetes, we struggle to bring their glycated haemoglobin level within control. We often have to use additional medications which add to the cost as well as to the possible side effects. Here are two examples, where, without changing any medicine, and by using simple behavioural modification tools, we were able to bring about profound changes leading to normalization of glycated haemoglobin levels.

This also applies in other medical situations. About a year ago, an elderly lady came to see me. She normally used to walk into my room, but on this occasion, she was brought in a wheelchair. When I asked her, I found out that she had arthritis and the pain in the joints prevented her from walking. At the end of the consultation, I casually remarked to her that if she wanted to see me next time, she would have to walk into my room without any support and definitely not come in a wheelchair. A few months passed and I forgot about this incident. When she came for her next review with me, she proudly walked in and said, 'I have done it, doctor.' For a moment, I could not understand what she was trying to say. She then reminded me, 'Last time, you told me that if I come in a wheelchair you would not see me. Hence, I have been practising at home, to walk by myself and was able to get rid of my wheelchair. Here I am, doctor.' I was overjoyed. Once again it was reaffirmed that the human mind has tremendous potential. All it needs is a little coaxing. Different methods can be used in therapy and some of these may appear unscientific. They certainly do not teach us these techniques in medical college. But more often than not, miraculous results can be obtained by using these unconventional but powerful behaviour-modification tools. And the best part is: they cost nothing!

Sometimes, it's not about achieving results but about doing what's right. As a spiritual person, I often come across situations where I have to make a decision about treating a patient based on modern science or spirituality. It's an ethical debate.

For about thirty years, I had been treating a woman who had done quite well until recently her health began to fall. She developed an enlargement-of-the-heart condition called diabetic cardiomyopathy where the heart not only becomes enlarged but also flabby. This means that it was unable to pump blood effectively. Although medicines are available for this, the only treatment is a heart transplant, which is not always feasible due to various constraints, including the availability of a donor heart.

The patient had been admitted to the hospital many times, and each time she recovered and went home. But this time when she came to see me, she had a very weak heart and needed emergency admission. She was not prepared for the admission and said she would rather die than get admitted in the hospital. I realized that she was terrified of being admitted into the ICU. This is always a fear among patients because of the anxiety-inducing sound of the ventilators, the constant beep of monitors and the overall atmosphere of fear. When I asked the patient what she was scared of, she said, between hurried breaths, that she was afraid of dying alone in a cold ICU. She therefore absolutely refused to get into the ICU, and the family sought a compromise with me and asked if she could be kept in an ordinary hospital room which would have oxygen but not other facilities like a ventilator.

This was a huge ethical decision to take. And when I consulted our ICU specialist, he ruled it out unequivocally. It was too risky, he said. I called her children aside and had a long chat with them. It was very clear that they had accepted that their mother was dying. She was acutely breathless and clearly suffering but she didn't want to go to the ICU. And it would have been inhumane to send her home.

At that point, I took the decision to keep her in an ordinary hospital room. It was the patient's intense desire, as well as that of her children. They wanted to be together in her last moments. We agreed that we would give it our best shot and see whether we could pull her out of her current situation. If that happened, it would be a miracle. On the other hand, if she succumbed, the family would find solace in the fact that they were with their mother during her last moments.

We admitted her into a hospital room and looked after her to the best of our ability. We even shifted a ventilator into her room. She made a transient recovery and was all smiles as her symptoms had been relieved and she was able to breathe. Later that night, when the children were singing her favourite bhajans, their mother passed away peacefully with a smile on her face, without any discomfort.

The children and the rest of the family were extremely grateful to me for allowing this and felt that their mother had been at total peace, without any fear, and had died while they were holding her hands. This was a very special moment for me because I had followed my conscience. The woman's last wish—of not dying alone in a cold, frightening ICU but peacefully with her children at her side singing her favourite songs when she took her last breath—had been fulfilled, too.

24

The Importance of Mentoring

One of the greatest values of mentors is the ability to see ahead what others cannot see and to help them navigate a course to their destination.

—John C. Maxwell, leadership expert, speaker and author

There's no one-size-fit-all guide to what constitutes success but a collection of things: how individuals feel about working in an organization, how the teams collaborate with each other, whether people find the right support at the workplace and whether they're repeatedly pushed to work better. Today, if we run fifty-two diabetes clinics across the country, a key reason for that success is an increased focus on helping people identify their talents and supporting them through the journey.

Our two-year residential fellowship in the diabetes programme has consistently helped us identify and hone new talents. These two years are especially beneficial as they give us sufficient time to not only train the resident doctors in diabetes but also to teach them patient handling and the art of medicine apart from the science of medicine. Many of them imbibe the traits they see in their teachers and apply them in their own practice.

An essential aspect of the training is to write adequate notes about the patient's condition. In both the outpatient and inpatient departments, doctors are taught to write notes, complete discharge summaries and check for completeness and errors. Unfortunately, many hospitals neglect this step. I am very strict about this and train doctors to be accurate in their findings whenever they document their clinical findings. The benefits become apparent only later.

I once noticed that one of the fellows took detailed, elaborate notes. He clearly had a talent for writing, which seemed to be far above that of the other fellows. One day, when I saw him write, I casually told him, 'I think you have the makings of a writer in you.'

The kind, encouraging words of seniors can often have a life-changing impact on young practitioners—and that's exactly what happened. After the fellow completed his course, instead of practising diabetes full-time, he took up pharmacovigilance (a field that involves the preparation of copious amounts of written records) and immersed himself in intensive research on drugs. In subsequent years, he rose through the ranks in his chosen field and won a lot of recognition.

Another aspect of the residential diabetes course is how it encourages students to unleash their hidden talents, such as public speaking. This works in many ways: it helps doctors improve their knowledge, get over stage fright and, importantly, become effective communicators.

About ten years ago, I noticed that one of our fellows was extraordinarily confident and clear in her presentation. I called her aside and told her, 'I think you have a talent for speaking; you should keep this up.' She was both surprised and pleased to hear this, and promised me that she would try her best. Over the years, I found that she was growing from strength to strength and being invited to speak, initially, at regional and, later, at national and international meetings. Everywhere she went, she made a huge impact, and would receive more invitations to speak. She continues to excel as a public speaker and popular medical teacher today.

Many such fellows have convinced me that if talent is spotted early and nurtured, people can climb to great heights and excel in their professions. It's all about mentoring and providing the right atmosphere for our students and juniors.

But if I am able to mentor someone today, it's because people took the time and effort to mentor me. In 1976, when I was in the final year of MBBS, I would dutifully read *Joslin's Diabetes Mellitus*, a book which my fellow classmates were not even aware of. One day, when I was reading a particular portion of this text, I saw a radiograph (X-ray) that immediately caught my attention, because I had picked up a similar case in my father's clinic. It was an X-ray of the pelvis, showing calcification of the vas deferens—a tiny muscular tube in the male reproductive system. I wrote to the author of the particular chapter, Dr Stephen Podolsky, who was from Boston and told him that I had seen a similar case and was interested in learning more from him. Dr Podolsky immediately wrote back and encouraged me to perform a small study looking at a series of male patients and seeing how many had calcification of the vas deferens. This proved to be a very simple study as all it needed was an X-ray of the pelvis. I studied 500 patients and reported the first prevalence study of calcification of the vas deferens from India as a clinical sign of diabetes. But while researching this, we also found something grievous. Those who had calcification of the vas deferens did not live very long as they also developed multiple other complications. And so we proposed that this was a sign of poor prognosis in people with diabetes. That is, if this sign was present, it indirectly indicated that the patient probably had multiple other—and possibly more serious—diabetes-related complications. When I wrote to Dr Podolsky with the results, he was extremely pleased that I had made the effort to follow up on his advice.

That year, the World Diabetes Congress was being held for the first time in India and the main event was in New Delhi, while several smaller satellite symposia of the main congress were being held in various other cities in India. My father was organizing the Chennai edition, with a satellite symposium on the subject of pancreatic diabetes. I told my father about my correspondence with Dr Podolsky and floated the idea of inviting him. Not only was Dr Podolsky pleased to arrive, he spoke passionately about the subject of secondary forms of diabetes and even mentioned my paper in his talk. He also spent quality time with me and encouraged me by saying he had never seen a medical student who was so passionate about research. He said that I would become a world leader in diabetology one day and would publish many research papers if I kept up the same level of passion.

After the conference, he proposed to my father that they write a textbook, which covered not only the proceedings of the Chennai satellite symposium but also collaborate with other scientists to get additional chapters for the book. This led to the birth of a book titled *Secondary Diabetes: The Spectrum of the Diabetic Syndromes* by Podolsky and Viswanathan. To date, this is the only book that discusses the form of diabetes where a secondary cause is known, like stones in the pancreas or cancer of the pancreas, among other causes.

Dr Podolsky was a very busy man. He didn't need to spend time with me but he did. Throughout his stay, his simple words of positive encouragement, his outlook and his gentle mentoring solidified my interest in diabetes. We later visited Dr Podolsky at his centre in Boston and this helped to further strengthen our ties.

Two months prior to the scheduled Chennai symposium, Dr C. Gopalan, the former director of the National Institute of Nutrition, Hyderabad, and the director general of the Indian Council of Medical Research had invited my father to deliver a lecture at a similar satellite symposium on nutrition and diabetes which was to be held in Hyderabad. But merely a couple of days before the symposium, a senior professor who was helping my father organize the Chennai event backed out due to a personal emergency. As he had too much to do for the Chennai symposium, my father decided against going to Hyderabad.

But instead of simply pulling out, my father gave me a shocker. He asked me to deliver the speech in his place. To say that I was flabbergasted would be an understatement. I was furious with my father for sending me like this at such short notice with no preparation and my final-year MBBS exams just round the corner. But before I could react, I was on a flight to Hyderabad.

My father, good-naturedly, also called the chairman of that particular session where I was scheduled to speak and informed him about my predicament. And here I was, standing in front of medical stalwarts from around the globe, many of whom I had admired for so long. To them, I would have looked like a weary, sleep-deprived medical student, had I not been able to master the gist of my father's talk on the flight to Hyderabad.

I must have delivered a great talk, because as soon as I finished, the audience gave me a standing ovation. Terrified at first, I also managed to defend a barrage of questions with relative ease. And when I finished the conference and came out, I found myself mobbed by people. I was pleasantly surprised when the ICMR director general, Prof. C. Gopalan, paid me some rich compliments. It was my first meeting with the great man who considered a living legend in the field of nutrition and the first medical doctor from India to be elected a fellow of the Royal Society in the UK. Years later, Prof. Gopalan invited me to deliver one of the most prestigious lectures in the medical field, the C. Ramachandran Memorial Lecture, which had been instituted in his late son's name. It was a profound privilege for me to deliver this lecture; still later, I also had the good fortune to meet the great man when he celebrated his hundredth birthday!

When I returned home, my father confided in me that the chairman of the session, Prof. B.B. Tripathy, had been so impressed with my talk that he had decided to closely mentor me in the years to come. Not only diabetes, Prof. B.B. Tripathy taught me ethics, what to publish and what not to publish. Quite simply, he taught me the art of scientific publishing. And it all started with a talk that I was not even meant to deliver!

But just like the students I would mentor later in my life, I had been a sincere student, always eager to learn more; that's what impressed my mentors, from Prof. Tripathy to Dr Podolsky. Most notably, I was proactive. Merely seeing an X-ray in a textbook propelled me to write to Dr Podolsky, establish a friendship with him, which in turn led to his visit to India, to our visit to his centre in Boston and culminated with us penning a famous textbook on secondary diabetes together. If I had not seen that photograph, or had not written to Dr Podolsky, none of this would have come to fruition. Now, when I look back, I marvel at how eager I was to learn and it was that enthusiasm that introduced me to people who would help me find success. Mentors might find you anywhere—but are you prepared for their guidance?

25

Using the Power of Positive Thinking in Healing

When you want something, all the universe conspires in helping you to achieve it.

—Paulo Coelho, Brazilian author

Several years ago, a twenty-six-year-old girl was admitted under my care. This girl had type 2 diabetes and her blood sugar levels, although uncontrolled, were not markedly elevated. She had developed a dental infection and, due to this, her blood glucose levels had gone up. It is well known that infections and blood glucose levels share a vicious cycle. Thus, an increase in blood glucose levels shows a predisposition to infections and, conversely, infections increase blood glucose levels.

Treating one condition, then, helps improve the other. I planned a simultaneous treatment for the dental infection and the control of her diabetes. She was admitted to the hospital and was being treated with insulin and anti-diabetic tablets for diabetes and antibiotics for the dental infection. I expected that over the next couple of days, her blood glucose levels would stabilize and then a dental surgeon would be able to step in and cure her dental infection—if necessary, by performing a small dental procedure. But soon after the admission, she shocked me by saying, 'Doctor, I will not survive this. I am going to die.' I was taken aback. Nothing in her clinical condition warned me of any mortal danger and hence I assured her that she would recover and soon be home.

But she persisted: 'No, doctor, I will not survive. I will die soon.' I tried to reason with her and told her that she had a simple infection which was easily controllable and reprimanded her for her morbid thoughts. Her blood sugars initially dipped but after a couple of days, they started rising and her infection, too, started spreading rapidly. She developed severe cellulitis (an inflammation of subcutaneous connective tissue) in what is referred to as 'the dangerous area of the face', as, from there, it can easily spread to the brain. Within the next twenty-four hours, it did spread to the brain, leading to a severe brain abscess and then ultimately to coma. Despite the best treatment, her condition continued to deteriorate and, twelve days after she had predicted that she would not survive, she passed away.

This incident had a profound impact on me because when the patient first told me she would not survive, she definitely was not in a serious condition at the time. She was fully conscious and the infection was in its early stages. No doctor could have predicted that the illness would take such a serious turn. Since then, I have often asked myself: *How did this girl know that she would die?* Was it intuition or did her thoughts lead to the rapid worsening of her condition? If it was the latter, what was the exact mechanism through which her negative thoughts caused the progression of the disease, ultimately leading to her death? I am afraid that even after all these years, I do not have the answers to these questions. But as this was in the early years of my practice, it did influence me a great deal. I began to believe that there is a very strong *mind–body connection*.

Several years later I would have to apply my knowledge of the mind–body connection to my own self. When I lost my wife, Rema, not only did I lose my partner but also my best friend and soulmate. Her departure created a huge vacuum in my life, and at that time, I didn't even have my spiritual guru to fall back on, because thirty days after Rema's demise, my guru, Bhagawan Sathya Sai Baba, left his physical body, too. I was at the ashram, completely shattered, but fulfilling my duty of sitting by my guru's coffin as hundreds of thousands of disciples paid their respects as well. In a span of thirty days, I had lost not only my wife and life partner but also my beloved guru—and no amount of consolation seemed enough.

It was the most difficult time of my life and only through intense prayer, pranayama and yoga was I able to prevent myself from falling apart. Books, too, helped me get through this difficult period. One that is etched in my mind is *The Autobiography of a Yogi* by Paramahansa Yogananda. In Chapter 43, Yogananda talks about how his guru was resurrected and appeared to him in flesh and blood and explained to him what happens after the soul leaves the body. I derived great solace after reading this and it gave me the strength to grieve. Bhajans at Prasanthi Nilayam, the abode of peace, the ashram where my guru lived all his life, helped too.

I then decided that I needed to move on and started planning my future. My daughter and I drew ambitious plans for the expansion of the hospital and for increasing research activities. She insisted that I travel to places that I wanted to go to but had never found the time for. The past was behind me and now, powered by positive thinking, I was looking ahead and starting again to immerse myself in my work. My physical health, too, became a priority and I increased my exercise and sleep. This meant that my energy levels soared and I was able to achieve more than I had in previous years. Most importantly, I spent more time with my immediate family—

my daughter, son-in-law and grandson—and they helped fill the twin voids in my life to a large extent.

By then, I was also encouraging my patients to imbibe these key life-altering practices such as pranayama or positive thinking in their lives. But I didn't know if diabetes or its complications could be reversed by the power of positive thinking. I was eager to test my hypothesis. Shortly after, I saw a patient who had moderate damage to his kidneys, which were leaking a large amount of albumin in the urine. At this stage, the condition usually deteriorates and the chances of getting back to normal are quite bleak. His brother also had a kidney disease due to diabetes which had in fact progressed, and so he was afraid that, like his brother, his disease would also worsen.

After we started the treatment, I would spend some time talking to him, telling him that together we would work to make his kidneys normal again. I then taught him a small mantra; I asked him to look at his reflection in the mirror, every morning, and say the following words twenty times: *My kidney will become normal.* I wanted to check whether a chronic medical illness like kidney disease can be slowed or reversed by positive reinforcement.

Three months later he returned for his review and, when the results of his various tests arrived, I was ecstatic to note that his kidney was functioning normally. The albuminuria which he had earlier had disappeared.

One can argue that this was the spontaneous reversal of an early kidney disease, or that the prescribed medicines had worked. I agree that this is entirely possible and the repeating of the mantra probably had nothing to do with the reversal in the disease. But one can also argue that the positive reinforcement worked by way of behaviour modification and better adherence to the medicines, and this helped in the healing process. Again, entirely possible. While there is no way I can scientifically prove whether the positive reinforcement worked, the fact remains that the patient was cured.

Moreover, research has shown that those with a positive bent of mind, or optimists, are more proactive and tend to have better cardiovascular health and a stronger immune system. The question is: How are optimists able to remain positive? Optimism is a trait that can be learnt by consciously shifting your focus and perspective to pleasant thoughts. The more vigorously and consciously we change our day-to-day bad scenarios to positive ones, the more we train our brains to alter our reactions to position motions, which has healing power. The brain is also intimately connected to the body through the nerves. Various neurochemical factors, endocrine hormones, cytokines and pro- and anti-inflammatory molecules also exist in the body. Is it implausible that positive vibes affect this orchestra of biological factors in a positive way and accelerate healing? What about negative thoughts pushing one deeper into the disease state? Still, the exact process by which the mind controls susceptibility or recovery from illness remains a mystery and is a fertile field for future research.

For my part, I encourage all my patients—from those suffering from intractable migraines and headaches, body pain, abdominal pain, kidney disease or painful diabetic neuropathy—to support their healing with positive reinforcement and allow the power of the mind to help them achieve the desired results. And I continue to be amazed by the results obtained.

26

The Power of the Subconscious Mind

All that we are is the result of what we have thought.

—Gautama Buddha, the founder of Buddhism

When I was growing up, I idolized Dr Frederick Banting—the person who discovered insulin. I might have never received formal instruction from him but his stories demonstrated a sense of grit that few could match. His keen interest in and passion for diabetes came from his mother, who suffered from the disease, and ever since, he wanted to find a cure for it. Banting threw himself into diabetes research. His unwavering focus on finding a cure for diabetes filled his working hours. But his nights were not spared either. One night, frustrated, he went to bed but had a disturbed sleep. Around 2 a.m., he got up from his bed and, half asleep, scribbled in a notebook, the following words—*Diabetus, Ligate pancreatic ducts of dogs, keep dogs alive: till acini degenerate leaving islets, try to isolate the internal secretion of these to relieve glucosuria*—and went back to sleep.

Banting continued doing this: he would wake up the following morning and read his notes scribbled in a half-asleep state. This led to his famous dog experiments with Charles Best, who then was a young medical student. Their work would eventually lead to the historical discovery of insulin. Banting's relentless pursuit to cure diabetes seeped into his subconscious mind. And his subconscious mind gave him the solution that changed the face of diabetes forever. Few other stories can be as demonstrative of the power of the subconscious mind as this: that insulin was discovered not by a diabetologist or an endocrinologist but by a surgeon who did not even spell diabetes correctly in the notes he scribbled when half asleep.

Ever since Sigmund Freud helped us understand the mind and its three levels of awareness, or consciousness—the conscious mind, the subconscious mind and the unconscious mind—we know that every thought that occurs in the conscious state, if sensed to be true by the brain, is sent to the subconscious mind.

In his famous book *Blink: The Power of Thinking without Thinking*, Malcolm Gladwell, talks about the power of trusting our instincts. The message is clear: the more you develop your intuition, the stronger it gets. It's difficult to explain how intuition works but it almost always does.

When I meet my patients, I am able to divide them into those who have a sense of intuition and faith and are able to incorporate positive thinking in their life and those who don't. The former are often labelled fortunate; but it's not that they're merely relying on luck—they have faith and self-confidence. Srinivasa Ramanujan, the world-renowned Indian mathematician, declared that he received the mathematical inspirations for his formulae by praying to Goddess Namagiri, the Hindu goddess of creativity. We can also interpret his faith as his deep intuition and connection to his subconscious mind which helped him tap into intelligence from sources beyond human comprehension. Together, faith and self-confidence can brew magic. Ramanujan said, 'An equation for me has no meaning unless it expresses a thought of God.'

Intuitions, impulses, hunches or a strong idea—we often refer to these as our 'gut feeling'. Many great scientists and artists have skilfully tuned in to their subconscious minds to create and generate new ideas. Albert Einstein, for example, played the violin and the piano between his work. Music helped him concentrate when he was thinking about his theories. He would strike a chord or two, fully engrossed in his thoughts, and then quickly jot down his ideas and get back to his study. To quote Einstein, 'A new idea comes suddenly and in a rather intuitive way. But intuition is nothing but the outcome of earlier intellectual experience.'

In the early years of my practice, a fifty-year-old gentleman came to consult me for a routine diabetes check-up. He was a well-known, deeply respected industrialist, with an impressive social standing. During the check-up, I detected that he had mild renal (kidney) damage. He was blissfully unaware of this, although his tests a few months ago had also shown elevated serum creatinine levels. It therefore came as a rude shock to him when I mentioned to him that he had diabetic kidney disease. He then made a strange request: 'Doctor, I am now fifty years told. I want to be alive till I am seventy-five. So for the next twenty-five years, you have to help me to keep going. It is my fervent wish that I should not undergo dialysis or transplantation for the next twenty-five years. Can you help me, doctor?'

This was a rather tall order, for we know that diabetic kidney disease is a relentlessly progressive condition, and once renal failure sets in, it leads to a downward spiral. In most cases, patients reach end-stage renal disease (ESRD) within five to ten years. And in ESRD, only two treatments are available: dialysis or the transplantation of the kidneys. I assured the gentleman that I would do my best and told him that if he cooperated by controlling his diabetes and blood pressure well, we would work together to fulfil his dream. He promised me that he would come for his check-up as often as needed. Thus started a long journey with this patient who, in the process, became a very close friend of mine.

What's noteworthy in this case is that the man was extremely disciplined and would follow all the instructions meticulously. He would visit me regularly and maintain the best possible sugar and blood pressure levels through a careful diet, exercise and medicine programme. As a result, for several years, his renal parameters remained relatively stable, without too much of deterioration. In fact, if his serum creatinine level (a marker of renal function) went up, to, say, 3.5 mg/dl, he would say, 'Doctor, when I come back next month, it will be 2.5 mg/dl.' Initially, I didn't take him seriously, as there are no medicines or lifestyle measures to *reduce* serum creatinine levels. The best one can hope to achieve is *maintain* the same level. But when the man would return for his next visit, the creatinine levels would have fallen, just as he had predicted. It was all quite eerie. When I questioned him as to how he managed to do this, he gave a remarkable response: 'By sheer willpower and prayer.' He had a deep and unshakable faith in God and truly believed that prayer would improve his clinical condition. Time and again, over the next few years, I saw this happen. In this manner, twenty-five years passed, and when he turned seventy-five, he was still off dialysis and transplantation, just like he had desired when he first saw me.

What was this gentleman doing differently? In reality, he was allowing his subconscious mind to do the task. He was tapping into the power of his subconscious mind—not for creative inspiration but to live a healthy life. The subconscious mind faithfully listens to the thoughts that are fed to it by the conscious mind. And so feeding it positive thoughts about health, love and peace can help normalize body functions. The man knew and habitually practised thinking about good health and reaffirming to himself that he was fine and healthy. This was eventually passed on to the subconscious mind, which in turn improved his health.

My experience with this patient left me almost incredulous, but it has convinced me that there's something that goes on beyond what we know of medicine today. He is a living example of how discipline, positive thinking, willpower and prayer, in addition to medicines, can keep renal failure at bay for nearly three decades. And he is not the only one who has shown me that. Even in this day and age, medical miracles do happen.

27

The Importance of Committing to Yourself

It's determination and commitment to an unrelenting pursuit of your goal—a commitment to excellence—that will enable you to attain the success you seek.

—Mario Andretti, Italian-born
American automobile-racing driver

When we were in medical college, four of my close friends and I had a heart-to-heart discussion about what we would do with our lives. One of them, Mohan Kameswaran, said that he would become an ENT surgeon, following in his illustrious father's footsteps. The second, Nandagopal, said that he would become a surgeon, specializing in plastic surgery, again continuing the work pioneered by his father. The third friend, Mayilvahanan (Mayil), said he would take up orthopaedic surgery following, once again, in his well-known father's footsteps. And the fourth friend, Naresh, said he would become a cardiothoracic (heart and lung) surgeon, as he had recently been influenced by the lives of the famous American cardiac surgeons Michael DeBakey and Denton Cooley after reading their inspiring life stories.

Finally, it was my turn. I told my friends that I wanted to become a diabetes specialist and a researcher in diabetes, and added that my ambition was to publish the highest numbers of research papers in the world by a practising diabetologist. My friends smiled in disbelief and one of them remarked that it was not good to have so much ambition. If the bar is set too high, he said, it can hurt if you don't make it. But I held my ground and maintained that there was nothing wrong in dreaming big. I must admit that at the time I was influenced by the legendary boxing champion Muhammad Ali (born Cassius Clay), who had famously stated: 'I am the greatest.' Some of my friends thought that it was sheer arrogance that got Ali to make such a declaration. I thought that by making this statement, Ali was merely telling the world—and, more importantly, himself—that it was possible for him to become the greatest boxer ever. Ali did indeed go on to defeat some of the greatest boxers of his time, and is remembered, even today, as one of the greatest boxers the world has ever seen. I believe that it is not wrong to make such statements (particularly to oneself), because by doing this, you are sowing the seeds of self-confidence and preparing yourself to become the best in whatever field of work you set out to specialize in.

Is there any such thing as a great diabetologist? Most doctors who treat diabetes merely get the blood sugars of their patient or, at best, their glycosylated haemoglobin in levels (a test of the three months' control of diabetes) under control—and that's their primary, and often only, target. Good diabetologists also look at other systems and check whether the blood pressure and lipids are under control. Those with a more holistic approach go one step further: they look at the complications of the disease by examining the eyes, kidneys, heart and feet, and see that they are all kept under control. Doing the latter on all patients is a formidable task, as it needs a full-fledged diabetes centre with multiple specialists. Few clinics or centres can offer or could afford such facilities. In my case, ever since I spoke about researching on diabetes, my commitment to the cause of the disease has been much more intense. My vision was not just to provide succour and comfort to patients with diabetes and help them get their disease under control, but to actually help them live a long and healthy life, despite diabetes. It's been this vision, which I consider larger than myself, that has driven me to keep going and work on large-scale initiatives on understanding diabetes and trying to prevent it.

In order to prevent diabetes, one has to understand the natural history of diabetes. Before one develops the signs and symptoms of diabetes—the so-called clinical diabetes stage—one passes through the stage of 'pre-diabetes'. This is the stage between normal glucose levels and frankly diabetic glucose levels.

Even before this stage, there is another when the glucose levels are normal—the stage of normal glucose tolerance (NGT). At this stage of NGT, the risk factors for diabetes are already at work: overweightedness or obesity, physical inactivity, unhealthy eating and stress. These 'diabetogenic' factors eventually push the individual through to the stage of pre-diabetes and finally to the clinical-diabetes stage. If uncontrolled, even at the latter stage, one can move to the last stage of complications of diabetes. At this stage, reversal is no longer possible.

All these stages occur slowly over a period of years in an individual's life. Nature therefore gives one enough time to make the proper lifestyle changes to prevent NCDs like diabetes, hypertension, heart disease and even some cancers related to the above metabolic diseases. However, if we are to succeed, we have to start early—right from childhood. Today, more and more children are becoming obese. It is well known that childhood obesity leads to adult obesity and then to diabetes and other NCDs. Thus, the writing on the wall in clear: if we want to prevent obesity and eventually diabetes, we have to start early.

With this in mind we started a huge programme to prevent obesity in children. Through the Obesity Reduction and Awareness and Screening of Noncommunicable Diseases through Group Education in Children and Adolescents (or ORANGE) project, we reached out to 22,000 children in over 100 schools in Chennai, both government and private, where we taught them the importance of healthy eating, physical exercise and the overall need to prevent or treat obesity. The project was a huge success and led to an improvement in the lifestyles and health of thousands of children.

One can practise the prevention of diabetes at these three levels: primary, secondary and tertiary. For example, if the eye is already affected, we try to prevent the loss of vision in the eye, or if vision is already affected in one eye, we try to prevent the other eye from going blind. This is called 'tertiary prevention'. In 'secondary prevention', people who have diabetes, but don't have any complications as yet, are helped to stay that way, so that they never develop any complications and thus live a long, healthy life. In 'primary prevention', we focus on the pre-diabetes stage to prevent the onset of diabetes itself by diet, exercise and weight reduction in those who are overweight.

The next question one might logically ask is: Can diabetes actually be prevented? In collaboration with Prof. K.M. Venkat Narayan and his colleagues at Emory University, Atlanta, we conducted a large diabetes-prevention programme called the Diabetes Community Lifestyle Improvement Programme (D-CLIP). We gave those with pre-diabetes sixteen lessons in lifestyle modification, diet and exercise. After conducting a large study on this programme, we found that we were able to prevent diabetes in about 30 per cent of the people with pre-diabetes—a huge number, if you think about the 80 million people with pre-diabetes in India to whom these results directly apply.

While community studies and initiatives are important, lifestyle modification needs large-scale awareness. With this in mind, we started a massive Let's Defeat Diabetes (LDD) programme, which involved the public in Chennai, Bengaluru and Hyderabad. This has been supported by both members of the community as well as celebrities like the cricketing legend Anil Kumble and the infrastructure development tycoon G.V.K. Reddy, among many others.

It's been my lifelong dream to help prevent diabetes, and early in life I realized that it's only commitment to research and on-ground activities that will help me do that. This is also why I work with the government through the National Programme for Prevention and Control of Diabetes, Cardiovascular Diseases and Stroke (NPDCS) and several other programmes. The focus is on last-mile outreach and ensuring that people focus on weight loss and improving physical activity. This is done in schools, workplaces and the overall community in several districts of India.

Each of these campaigns have been conducted over a span of several decades and help me inch closer and closer to my vision of helping Indians with diabetes live longer and healthier lives. If you ask me how I did it, it's a combination of various factors, but one that I particularly believe helps is the power of committing to a task and consistently reaffirming its value to yourself. Do it by making a list where you note down everything you desire and aim to achieve, or by using the sheer power of the mind and commitment to chase it.

As for my friends, who were discussed at the beginning of this chapter, they all continue to be committed to their fields of

chosen practice, as prominent doctors and committed members
of the fraternity, and all of them have become what they proposed
they would become, when we were still hardly out of our teens—
outstanding surgeons and world leaders in their own chosen
speciality of surgery.

28

Success Stories of People with Diabetes

I was determined to share my positive approach and not let diabetes stand in the way of enjoying my life.

—Paula Deen, American
TV personality and cooking-show host

Many people with diabetes believe that because of their illness, they cannot achieve their ambitions. Of the two most common forms of diabetes, type 2 and type 1, the former can be treated with tablets, diet and exercise, although some individuals may need insulin at some point in their life. Type 1 diabetes, on the other hand, is a more severe form of the disorder where insulin injections are needed from the beginning, and often several times a day, in order to maintain good health. I have seen that when people develop type 1 diabetes (or even type 2 diabetes, for that matter), they often tend to give up. Their family also thinks that they are doomed to a life of mediocrity, devoid of any ambitions or success.

Doctors, too, unknowingly, reinforce this mindset. We were taught as students that if somebody is fifty years old and has had diabetes for twenty years, their arteries and blood vessels would be seventy years old. We therefore recognize what's referred to as the 'chronological age', which is the actual age of the patient, and the 'biological age', which is the age of the arteries. In the case of people with diabetes, almost every study has shown that diabetes decreases the lifespan of an individual. Statistics show that in both men and women between seven to eight years of life are lost due to diabetes. Currently, the average lifespan of an Indian is sixty-seven years for males and sixty-nine years for females. Hence, for Indians with diabetes, one would expect that the average lifespan would be around sixty years for both males and females. By this calculation, one would assume that it would be almost impossible to find an elderly person with diabetes in India. Only 0.001 per cent of India's population today are nonagenarians, that is aged ninety years or above. Hence, finding a ninety-year-old person with diabetes in India would be an absolutely rarity.

While these statistics are well established, they're not necessarily true, and moreover, there are a lot of exceptions to the rule. Over the last few years, we have been noticing at our centre that our patients with diabetes, presumably due to better control, are living longer and longer. In 2013, I published a paper to show that patients with type 2 diabetes could live for forty or fifty years despite their diabetes. This paper was published in the prestigious American journal *Diabetes Care* and became a landmark paper. My colleagues and I were pleased that we as Indians were the first to report on the long-term survival of patients with type 2 diabetes.

After we had submitted the paper, Dr William Cefalu, then the editor of *Diabetes Care*, visited me in Chennai. Dr Cefalu told me that he was delighted to receive our paper and wanted to learn more about the survival among people with type 2 diabetes. Dr Cefalu then suggested that we have, as a control group, patients who were 'non-survivors', that is, had not survived for forty years. I mentioned to him that this would take time, as we would have to painstakingly match the 'survivors' and 'non-survivors' from our large electronic records. He gave us additional time to do it, and once we were done, we submitted the paper again to the journal. The paper was an instant hit—and was the first in the world to demonstrate the long-term survival of patients with type 2 diabetes of more than forty years duration.

In fact, when I received the Harold Rifkin Award for Distinguished International Service in the Cause of Diabetes from the American Diabetes Association, Dr Cefalu was present at the ceremony. I walked up to him and asked him whether he remembered me. Dr Cefalu smiled and said, 'Why do you think you are receiving this award?' By then, Dr Cefalu was the chief scientific officer of the association and, despite his high position, he hadn't forgotten my paper in his journal. 'That paper of yours was definitely one of the highlights of your career,' he said. I agreed. I was humbled to receive the award, and even more so because I was the first diabetologist from India to have been chosen for the award.

However, in that study we did not take the age of the patients into consideration—only the duration of diabetes. Only recently have we started looking at our electronic medical records again to see how many patients lived very long lives. This time, our study showed that 325 of our patients with type 2 diabetes had survived beyond ninety years of age. This meant that if one applied the formula taught by our teachers, the biological age of these patients was unbelievably long. By now, I have several patients who have crossed ninety-five years of age and are approaching their hundredth birthday. I have also seen my first patient with diabetes cross the coveted hundred-year birth-anniversary mark. This man was the former vice chancellor of two universities and has had diabetes for almost sixty years. This means his biological age would be 160 years!

It's perhaps time to relook at some of the old fundamental teachings regarding diabetes, as we are repeatedly proving them wrong. But the question is: Why are some people able to do it and not others?

Some real champions of diabetes, especially people with type 1 diabetes, have had extraordinary success despite the disease. Gary Hall Jr is an American swimming champion who represented the United States at three Olympic Games and won a total of ten Olympic medals—five gold, three silver and two bronze. But Hall's story is truly an inspirational one. Gary Hall's father, Gary Hall Sr, also took part in three Olympics as a swimmer. His maternal uncle and his maternal grandfather were swimming champions as well. Coming from a family of world-class swimmers, Gary Hall Jr's ambition, from childhood, was to win an individual Olympic gold medal in swimming. In the first Olympics that he participated in, the 1996 Olympic Games in Atlanta, Hall won the team relay gold medal, but he could not win the individual gold, as the Russian swimmer Alexander Popov beat him, and he had to settle for the silver medal.

Hall was determined to return in form for the 2000 Olympic Games in Sydney and try again for the gold. But a year before the games, Hall was diagnosed with type 1 diabetes. He was told by his doctors that he would never be able to participate in competitive swimming again. Hall took a short break from swimming as the diagnosis had devastated him. But he decided to give it his best shot and soon went back to serious training. He eventually took part in the 2000 Sydney Olympics, where he won the gold medal in the individual 50 metres freestyle, in addition receiving to gold and silver medals in the team relays, along with a bronze medal. Not content with this, Hall continued to train and came back for the 2004 Olympics Games in Athens, where he again won the gold medal in the 50 metres freestyle. At twenty-nine, Hall became the oldest American male Olympic swimmer to win a gold medal. At the age of thirty-three, Hall tried again to participate in the 2008

Olympics, but this time he was disqualified after finishing fourth. He was, however, inducted into the US Olympics Hall of Fame. It is remarkable that after he developed type 1 diabetes, Hall was able to improve on the silver medal he won at the Atlanta Olympics (when he *did not* have diabetes) to win the gold medal at the Sydney Olympics (when he *did* have type 1 diabetes). Hall later became a spokesman for children with type 1 diabetes. He would take part in international conferences on diabetes as a guest speaker and motivate patients. I had the good fortune of meeting Gary Hall Jr at one of these diabetes conferences and found him to be truly inspiring and a role model for everyone with type 1 diabetes.

The winner of the Miss America Contest in 1999, Nicole Johnson, is another spokesperson for type 1 diabetes. When Nicole was diagnosed with type 1 diabetes at the age of nineteen, she was told that she would not be able to have a career or become a mother. But Nicole had other ideas. She took the bold decision of participating in the pageant wearing the insulin pump that she had to continuously sport to control her diabetes. She even publicly declared that she had type 1 diabetes and, without any inhibitions, pointed to the pump she was wearing. History was made when Nicole Johnson was crowned Miss America and became the first woman with diabetes to win the beauty contest. This was a great victory, not only for Nicole but also for all diabetes patients and insulin-pump users. She is also a mother now, proving doctors who told her she couldn't become a biological mother totally wrong.

In 2007, we received an email stating that Nicole Johnson was visiting India and that she was keen to see our diabetes centre in Chennai and interact with children with type 1 diabetes. We arranged a special meeting for her and Nicole spent time talking to, and motivating, children with type 1 diabetes and posing for photographs with them. She was truly an inspiration for the children.

The famous Pakistan cricketer and former captain of the Pakistan cricket team, Wasim Akram, is another great example of a diabetes champion. Wasim's career was at its peak and he had already taken about 250 wickets, when he was diagnosed with type 1 diabetes, at the age of thirty. Some of his doctors told him he would never be able to play professional cricket again. Wasim went on to prove all his critics, doctors and detractors wrong. He took another 250 wickets and ended with a record haul of 500 wickets in cricket, the second 250 wickets coming *after* he developed type 1 diabetes. All this was achieved while he continued to take insulin injections several times a day to battle his type 1 diabetes. He also actively involved himself in awareness campaigns for the disease.

Wasim visited us in Chennai and participated in a mega awareness programme on diabetes for school children with type 1 diabetes. What I really liked about Wasim was that he does not hide the fact that he has the disease. When I dined with him, I saw that he proudly displays his insulin pen on the dining table at restaurants and takes his insulin shots, when required, in full public view. He is a shining example of how, with willpower, one can overcome any obstacles or hurdles in one's life.

What's the one thing that's common to all these heroes and others who live to the age of ninety and beyond? They are all self-disciplined. They have been looking after their health in general, and diabetes in particular, quite well. They come for timely check-ups three to four times a year, enjoy physical activity and take their medicines regularly.

In the case of my nonagenarian patients, none of them is athletic or a sportsperson but all follow some discipline in their diet. Most importantly, they have the willpower and a positive approach to life. And, in the bargain, their inspirational stories have made diabetologists and scientists rewrite textbooks and journals.

29

The Price One Pays to Maintain One's Integrity

Supporting the truth, even when it is unpopular, shows the capacity for honesty and integrity.

—Steve Brunkhorst, counsellor and coach

There are moments in life when your integrity is tested. You are compelled to wade through the troubling waters of accusations and malice, unsure if you will be able to prove your innocence. Several times in life I have borne the brunt of standing up for a cause, and each time, I have tried to withstand the ruthless examination as best as I possibly could.

In 2013–14, an anti-diabetic drug threw my life into disarray. There are several groups of anti-diabetic drugs, and one such group is called the thiazolidinediones (TZD), which is an extremely powerful group of drugs and are known as 'insulin sensitizers'. In type 2 diabetes (unlike in type 1 diabetes, where insulin deficiency is the main cause), the main deficiency in the body is the ineffective action of insulin. This pathophysiological defect is referred to as 'insulin resistance', and to tackle the defect, insulin sensitizers are the obvious drugs of choice.

For nearly fifty years, a drug called Metformin has been extensively and almost exclusively used to tackle the problem of insulin resistance. When the TZD group of drugs were developed, they were shown to reverse the problem of insulin resistance even more efficiently and thus they proved to be true insulin sensitizers. Naturally, scientists were very excited about this development. But along with the excitement came disappointment. A drug has to be approved in the multiple stages of a clinical trial before reaching the market. First, there is a preclinical testing where it is tested on animals (although many scientists, concerned about animal testing, are devising newer ways to test drugs). If the drug is toxic to animals, it is dropped. Human trials then start, with the first phase of testing being designed mainly to see if the drug is safe, that is, to check that there are no adverse effects. Once this stage is cleared, the drug goes through a proper drug-development programme through phases two and three of clinical trials where an increasing number of patients are tested. And once the safety and efficacy of the drug and dosage are determined, the drug manufacturer applies to various agencies like the Federal Drug Administration (FDA) in the US and others for approval. It is only after this elaborate and mandatory process that a drug can be finally marketed.

When the TZD group of drugs were being tested, they started failing relatively early in the drug-development stage. The initial members of this class of drugs like Ciglitazone, Darglitazone, Englitazone and several others failed in the process and had to be eliminated. Other drugs which were closely related to this class were withdrawn due to proven drug toxicity. Finally, one drug in this class, called Troglitazone, was approved in the US and introduced to the market. However, there were indications that there could be toxicity due to this drug as well and so very few countries introduced this drug domestically. The Drugs Controller General of India (DCGI) denied permission for the introduction of Troglitazone in the Indian market.

In the US, after Troglitazone was introduced, several deaths were reported due to liver toxicity. And within a short period of time, the drug had to be banned and removed from the US market. Then, shortly after, came the good news that two drugs in the class had been declared safe and were introduced in the market: Rosiglitazone and Pioglitazone. Diabetologists all over the world were relieved that finally two TZD drugs could be used. Most of my colleagues in India, and I, became avid users of both these drugs as we found them to be extremely effective in lowering high glucose levels. However, there were definite side effects of both the drugs such as weight gain, sometimes massive swelling of the feet, fluid overload in the body, heart failure and increased risk of diabetic eye disease, especially a condition called maculopathy which sees fluid accumulation in the eyes. Eventually, more serious complications such as fractures in the upper limbs in women were reported. Then came the final straw: according to a publication from the Cleveland Clinic, an American academic medical centre based in Cleveland, Ohio, Rosiglitazone was said to increase the risk of heart attacks. This led to the withdrawal of Rosiglitazone from several markets and eventually from India as well.

Thus, from the year 2010, the only drug of the TZD class which remained in the market was Pioglitazone, which all of us continued to use. Around this time, the first reports of a possible bladder-cancer risk associated with the use of Pioglitazone emerged. And several reports regarding this were published in the US, the UK, France, Germany and other countries around the world. And then it hit closer home. One of my patients who was on Pioglitazone developed bladder cancer. Pretty soon, I had two more cases. At this stage, as I had already read the reports coming in from various countries,

I checked with a few of my colleagues in India and several confirmed that they also had cases of Pioglitazone-associated bladder cancer. A systematic study could not be performed immediately. So, we, a group of four or five diabetologists from India, decided to publish eight cases of possible Pioglitazone-associated bladder cancer in the form of a 'Letter to the Editor' in the *Journal of the Association of Physicians of India*. We wanted to alert other physicians and Indian authorities about the possible side effects of Pioglitazone. In the US, by now, several thousand lawsuits had been filed. Indeed, lawyers in the US were encouraging people to sue the drug manufacturer.

Around this time, one of my patients who had developed bladder cancer threatened to sue me. This prompted me to write a letter to the DCGI, warning about the possible side effects of Pioglitazone. I also enclosed the available published literature on the subject. In June 2013, the Government of India suddenly announced a ban on Pioglitazone, which took many by surprise. And then it was discovered by the Indian pharma industry that I had written a letter to the DCGI. At that time, the Pioglitazone market was worth Rs 800 crore in India, and several companies were marketing it. In the country, several generic versions of all drugs are produced, and in the case of Pioglitazone, double- and triple-drug combinations containing the drug were being produced. Physicians were therefore confused as to which drug contained what molecule. I had seen prescriptions of physicians writing the names of three drugs and all of them contained Pioglitazone. This was an alarming situation considering the possible severe side effects of the drug.

Once the contents of my letter were revealed, the pharma industry came down on me heavily. I was accused of being paid by competing pharma firms for creating this controversy. Hate mail was arriving for me via social media and email. It was a dark period of my life.

The government soon set up a committee to investigate the matter, and I was contacted by them for my views. At that time, I made my position clear. I said that in my opinion the drug was an effective anti-diabetic drug but it had far too many side effects, of which possible bladder cancer was only one. Moreover, its use was totally unregulated. After getting opinions from several specialists and stakeholders, the ban on Pioglitazone was lifted after about four weeks. However, several rules were stipulated by the government and the authorities as to how it should be used. It was clearly recommended that in suspected cases of bladder cancer, or if the drug was found to be ineffective, it should be withdrawn immediately. Finally, the government also banned irrational combinations of anti-diabetic drugs in which Pioglitazone was included. Lower doses of the drug were also introduced to ensure safety. It was clear that if I hadn't raised the red flag, none of this would have happened and Pioglitazone would have continued to cause harm to many more people in India.

But this episode had also caused *me* considerable harm. A few competitors took this as an opportunity to tarnish my image. I was criticized widely by my colleagues on social media and other channels. It took more than two years for me to regain my self-confidence. By this time, all over the world, the popularity of the drug had begun to drastically come down. In the United States, where 40 per cent of all type 2 diabetes patients were using the drug in 2004, it came down to 4 per cent in a few years' time. Moreover, the drug manufacturer was asked to pay billions of dollars to settle lawsuits.

In India, too, there was a sharp decline in the drug's popularity. I had stopped using the drug for my patients after the first instance of side effects surfaced, and I stood my ground even as both my practice and character were maligned. But I didn't lose a single night's sleep, for I had done the right thing. I, as a conscientious doctor, in order to protect the rights and safety of my patients, had placed the available evidence in front of the concerned authorities. This had come at a steep personal cost but I was confident that the truth would clear me and restore my reputation. And it eventually did.

30

How Spirituality Enriched My Life

To walk the spiritual path is to continually step out into the unknown.

—Wallace Huey, spiritual coach and author

As a young boy, I was fascinated by what happens after death. This led me to question the meaning of life and to understand the 'force', which we call 'God', which governs and controls the whole world. Unlike other children of my age, I would do a lot of reading on this subject. I was attracted to saints, and I remember spending a few days at the Aurobindo Ashram in Pondicherry (now Puducherry) as a teenager. I also read a lot of the great spiritual leader Sri Aurobindo's writings, including his poems, as I was very interested in poetry in those days. I found the Aurobindo Ashram to be very peaceful and was particularly influenced by the Auroville concept of universal brotherhood. But even though I was impressed, my heart kept telling me that there was something else that I was searching for.

A couple of years later, I also visited the Sri Ramana Ashram, which was home to the modern sage and Advaita Vedanta master Ramana Maharshi, as I was quite influenced by him, his simplicity and the profound truths that he enunciated. I found this ashram also to be very peaceful. Similarly, I had visited the ashrams of a few other saints apart from regularly visiting various temples. While all this gave me a lot of solace and peace, my heart kept telling me that there was something else that I had not yet seen, something that was waiting for me. I remember reading a couple of books on Sri Sathya Sai Baba, including *Sai Baba: Man of Miracles* by Howard Murphet. However, while the book made an impression on me, it still did not have the impact that it would have on me a few years later, that is, in the year 1992.

One of the turning points in my life came after my marriage to Rema. My father-in-law, Sri K.V. Thankappan Nair, was an ardent Ayyappa devotee and was a 'guruswamy', as he had been going to Sabarimala on pilgrimage for almost forty years. After I entered this family, I also started going to Sabarimala every year during the 'Mandala' puja season. My father-in-law was also one of those involved in building the now famous Ayyappan temple at Mahalingapuram in Chennai, where, later, a Guruvayurappan temple was also added. Hence, regular visits to this temple also followed. For almost fifteen years thereafter, Lord Ayyappa became the main deity in our home and all our prayers were to Lord Ayyappa.

In March 1992, six months after we had set up our new centre, Rema and I went to Bangalore to attend a diabetes conference. I found out from someone that Bhagawan Sathya Sai Baba (or Swami or Baba, as we devotees call Him) was at His Whitefield ashram in Bangalore. I asked my good friend Dr Shyamsundar (Shyam, as we call him), who is also a diabetologist and an ardent Sathya Sai Baba devotee, whether it was possible to go for Swami's darshan the following day to Whitefield. Shyam immediately obliged.

Early the next morning, accompanied by Shyam, Rema and I set off to Whitefield. We had been told that Swami would be there. However, as we approached the Whitefield ashram, Shyam remarked that He had probably left because many devotees were seen returning from the ashram. If Swami was there, nobody would leave the ashram at that time. When it was confirmed that Baba was not there, Shyam asked us whether we still wanted to enter the ashram. We said, 'Yes, why not? Having come so far, let us at least enter the ashram and see what it looks like.' The moment I stepped into the ashram, something hit me like a thunderbolt. It is very difficult to describe what exactly that feeling was, but I remarked to my wife and Shyam: 'This is it.' Surprised, they asked me, 'What do you mean?' I replied, 'This is what I have been waiting for all my life.'

It is very difficult to describe this feeling in scientific terms. Looking back on this incident, I am surprised that even after reading books about Swami earlier, I did not get this feeling. But when I entered the Whitefield ashram, it was like love at first sight, when Baba was not even physically there! But I could feel His presence very intensely. I immediately went to the bookstall and bought some books on Baba, including another copy of *Man of Miracles*. This time, upon on reading it, I felt completely transformed, and the book had a profound effect on me. My wife and I soon started attending the bhajan sessions at Sundaram, Baba's headquarters in Chennai.

We were both very attracted to the discipline of the Sri Sathya Sai Seva Organization and the calm, serene and peaceful atmosphere inside Sundaram. Baba's simple but effective lessons, including the eight-most-important words which summarize His entire teachings so well—*Love All, Serve All; Help Ever, Hurt Never*—also attracted us to Him and His organization. Rema and I both started not only attending the spiritual sessions regularly but also reading books about Baba. Soon after that, Baba came to Chennai and we were both blessed to be able to get a darshan. I remember waiting in the queue from 3 a.m. so that we would be in the first row when we entered Sundaram after Nagar Sankirtan (the singing of bhajans as we walked through the streets) and thus get to be as near Baba as possible.

The sight of Baba standing on the first floor of Sundaram and raising His hands in benediction and blessing all the devotees, at dawn, as the sun was just rising, is an image which is indelibly etched in my mind. Little did I realize then, that a decade later Baba would appoint me a member of the Sri Sathya Sai Trust in Tamil Nadu and, shortly thereafter, elevate me to the position of convenor of the board of trustees of the trust. Eventually, I would be promoted to the highest position one could possibly reach in the Sathya Sai Organization and trust, as a member of the board at trustees of the Sri Sathya Sai Central Trust at Prasanthi Nilayam, Baba's main ashram in Puttaparthi in Andhra Pradesh. I might have received multiple laurels in my life, but I still consider these positions the greatest honours I have ever received.

31

Anything Is Possible Through Prayer

Once we surrender our mind to God completely, He will take care of us in every way.

—Bhagawan Sri Sathya Sai Baba, Indian spiritual guru

One of the most powerful and unforgettable memories of my childhood involve Kishore, a childhood friend of mine and a school junior. A few months after I had passed my seventh-standard exams and entered the eighth standard, Kishore approached me in school and asked me whether I could give him my seventh-standard history book titled *The March of Time*. Without thinking, I said, 'Yes, please come and take it from me this evening at 4.30 p.m. after school.' I then completely forgot about it.

At 4.30 p.m., promptly, Kishore came home and rang the bell and my house help informed me that he had arrived. I panicked because I did not have a clue where the book was! As it had been a few months since I had last used the book, I had no idea where I had kept it. I quickly searched for it in the usual places, but the book was nowhere to be found. By nature, I am a person who hates to break a promise made. Hence, I was terribly upset and did not know what to do. Kishore was waiting outside and I had no clue where the book was! I then decided to use God's help and sat down in prayer and meditation and prayed: *God, if it is true that You really do exist and that You are all powerful, please show me* now *where that book is, so that I can give it to Kishore.*

A few minutes must have passed and my mind was completely blank. As I sat in meditation, suddenly, I had a vision of *The March of Time* kept in the most unexpected place, in the electricity-meter room outside my house, and that too on a sack of charcoal!

In our house in Royapuram, there was a small room called the 'meter' room, since it was used by people from the Tamil Nadu Electricity Board to record the electricity-meter readings, every month, for billing purposes. That room was opened on only two occasions: firstly, for the meter recording and, secondly, to store a sack of charcoal. This was in the 1960s, when LPG gas cylinders were not in use. The vision of the book placed on the sack of charcoal was totally surprising, but it was so vivid in my mind, that I immediately went out, called Kishore and opened this room to check for the book. The book was right where I saw it in my mind! Right on top of the sack of charcoal. To this day, I have not been able to explain how the book got there. This was one of the first 'tests' that I put God through as a child and it instantly reinforced my faith that there indeed is a power which is beyond all of us, a power to which we can turn to for solace whenever we are in need.

Most of my prayers those days were for material things. For example, the intensity of the prayers would increase at the time of the examinations and during the time the results were due to be announced. God would be forgotten whilst I started enjoying life with storybooks, movies or sports.

When I was doing my MBBS at Madras Medical College, I was the captain of the athletics team and my favourite sport was shot-put. I used to practise every day after college in preparation for the inter-medical sports competition. During the competition, a few weeks later, I was in second place after five throws had already been completed, and only one last throw was left. Unfortunately, I had not yet reached even my personal best in the first five attempts. The person ahead of me, in first place, had thrown the shot (which is basically an iron ball), a clear 1 metre more than me, and it was farther than anything I had ever thrown in my life. With my one last throw left, I prayed to God, *God help me with this one last throw, where I will use your help and not rely on my strength alone; so please help me, God*. It was miraculous that my sixth and last throw went a clear 1 metre over the distance of the person who was in first place at that time. This was a distance I had never recorded in my life, either before or since. I was convinced that the particular throw on that day was not my effort alone but was enabled by the Divine. I came to realize at that time about the power of the Divine and how God can instantly respond to a prayer even for as silly or selfish a cause as winning an athletic event. I also realized the truth of the words of the poet Alfred Lord Tennyson: 'More things are wrought by prayer than this world dreams of.'

This incident, however, induces a lot of questions. How does all this work? Is it true that by praying you get extraordinary belief, which adds to your physical or mental strength? Is it truly a miracle that God works through you? I have no clue whatsoever. But I do believe that faith is a powerful force.

Critics and sceptics have argued with me when I tell this story to them and ask me, 'What if your opponent had also prayed the same way, what would God do in such circumstances?' This is a question to which I do not have an answer. I suppose, this is where the 'spiritual bank' explanation comes in. My spiritual guru, Bhagawan Sathya Sai Baba, taught us: *Whatever you have in your spiritual bank comes to you at your time of need*. This indeed may be the reason why some prayers are answered and others are not. As a scientist, it would of course be stupid of me to say that anyone can beat an Usain Bolt in a 100-metres race in the Olympics just on the strength of a prayer. However, incidents such as these are probably meant to strengthen one's faith and also to remind one that God's power is limitless and His love unconditional.

I can only thank Him for responding to my prayer whenever I have prayed to Him. Mahatma Gandhi has said, 'I cannot remember a single instance where God has not answered my prayer.' And I strongly echo that sentiment as well. If God does not give us something that we ask for, it is only because He felt that we are better off without it or that it is in our best interest not to get it at the time. Years later, we ourselves realize why He did not answer that prayer and we will in fact thank Him for it. After many years, I continue to be convinced that if you pray to God, most of your prayers will be answered.

32

True Love Is Eternal

True love is unchanging. It is Divine.

—Bhagawan Sri Sathya Sai Baba, Indian spiritual guru

On our wedding day, 7 February 1979, I presented Rema with a gold ring. Inside the ring I had the following words engraved, *Love Is Eternal.* I was inspired to write these words after reading a book of that name by Irving Stone, just before our wedding. Rema wore this ring till the end of her life.

In the first week of January 2011, a few months before Rema had passed away, a strange thing occurred. A police officer came to my clinic and wanted to see me. When I invited him in and asked him what the matter was, he said that I had been nominated for an award. I was a bit confused and asked him for more details. He said that I had been nominated for the Padma Shri (which is the fourth-highest civilian award conferred by the Government of India after the Bharat Ratna, the Padma Vibhushan and the Padma Bhushan, respectively). Individuals who are shortlisted for the Padma Shri normally have to undergo police verification as well as get clearance from the income tax department before the awards are announced.

I was slightly taken aback; I was not aware that I had been nominated for the Padma Shri. Later I learnt that a friend in Delhi had nominated me for it. Normally, the Padma Shri awards are announced to the press by the Government of India on 25 January, i.e. the day before Republic Day. And on Republic Day (26 January), the newspapers and media carry the details of the recipients of the various awards. On 23 January 2011, there was a doctor's conference in Chennai. One of my friends, who had got some information about my name being on the list for the Padma awards that year, announced to all my colleagues that I was likely to get the Padma Shri that year. To my great embarrassment, everyone started congratulating me.

Two days later, when the list of the Padma awardees was announced, my name was not there! I was highly embarrassed, as many of my colleagues had already congratulated me prematurely for this two days earlier. Rema learnt about this and asked me, 'Are you disappointed that you did not get the Padma Shri?' I told her, 'Look, Rema, firstly, I did not apply for it. Secondly, I am not bothered about these awards. You are more important to me, and this is not the time to think of these awards.' She then told me something which shook me right to my inner core. She said, 'Mohan, you *will* get the Padma Shri next year, and although I will not be there physically, I *will* somehow let you know that I am aware of you getting the award.' As the topic was getting rather disturbing for me, I immediately dismissed all further discussion and said, 'This is not the time to discuss these matters, and anyway all this is not important to me. Let's change the topic.'

On 25 January 2012, ten months after Rema's passing, I went to work as usual around 9 a.m. In my consultation room, I have the portraits of my guru, Bhagawan Sri Sathya Sai Baba, and Rema. Every day, I put fresh garlands of fragrant jasmine flowers on the two pictures. On that particular morning, I went into my room as usual, garlanded the portraits and sat down in my chair. Then something strange started happening. The garland on Rema's picture started shaking quite violently and fell down. This had never happened before. I put the garland back and returned to my seat. Immediately, the garland on my guru's picture also started shaking and fell down. Once again, I hung the garland on the photo. Now, it was time for the garland on Rema's picture to shake again and fall down. This happened six times over the next three hours. This was something that had never happened before—and hasn't occurred since. Even my secretary noticed the shaking garlands and rushed to see what was happening. A few hours later, I got a call from the Ministry of Home Affairs in Delhi, informing me that I had been awarded the Padma Shri. I turned to look at the pictures of Baba and Rema and, as if on cue, the shaking of the garlands stopped.

Rema had told me that I would get the Padma Shri the following year and had also promised me that she would let me know that she knows of this news, even if she is not there with me physically. That my guru's portrait was also shaking at the same time as hers held special significance for me. It was that rare moment in my life when I connected with divinity—and it was a humbling as well as a deeply emotional moment for me.

I consider myself exceptionally blessed to have received my guru's and my dear wife's blessings on the day when the Government of India honoured me with the Padma Shri. It taught me that loved ones can connect with us long after they have left their physical form. *Love is indeed eternal.*

Epilogue

That's all, folks. I have told my story as honestly as I could. So what's my take-home message?

First of all, decide whether you really want success or not. There is a price for everything in life, including success; you must be prepared to pay for it. Jealousy, pain, sleepless nights, going beyond your comfort zone, sacrifices, working harder and smarter all the time, raising the bar frequently, failures, frustrations—the list is endless for those who want success. Some decide early in life that it is not worth it—it is just not their cup of tea. They decide that a laid-back life is what suits them best, and they are fine with it. In other words, they are happy with whatever they are able to achieve within their zone of comfort.

But there are others who like to take risks, push the boundaries, set higher and higher targets for themselves and desire to establish a legacy not as impermanent as their time on this earth. I wrote this book keeping the latter in mind and thinking about how I could enrich people's journeys with stories of my own. The fact that you cared to pick up this book and read it shows that you belong to this group of people.

Ultimately, I believe that success is due to many factors. On the top of the list are the social circumstances in which you are placed in life. It was fate that led an aspiring writer and poet like me to take up something quite removed from romance and poetry and embrace the harsh realities of being a doctor, dealing squarely with life and death and sickness. The fact that at the tender age of eighteen, I got the opportunity to work in my chosen speciality—diabetes— and conduct research was also a matter of happenstance. But then success is also about seizing the opportunities which stare at us, and making full use of them.

I also learnt early in life that one can wear multiple hats: of a doctor, researcher, teacher, administrator, philanthropist and spiritual and motivational speaker. The important thing is to focus on the job at hand. In this book, I have tried to share what I think are the basic qualities needed for anyone to succeed: passion, focus, resilience, hard work, faith, the courage to dream big, peer pressure and support, sharing and collaboration with others and, above all, integrity. All these are essential ingredients if one were to write a recipe for success.

And, finally, remember that life comes full circle. With the writing of this book, the dreams of a romantic teenager who wanted to become a writer are also partially fulfilled. I hope you have enjoyed reading this book of my life as much as I have enjoyed living it and, even more, writing about it. Finally, I also hope that a few dreamy-eyed teenagers somewhere on this planet will be inspired by this book and that it helps them write their own success stories decades later.

Acknowledgements

Through this book, I might have given the impression that I romanticize workaholism, or a life that leaves little time for anything else other than work. This not entirely untrue, as during my earlier years as a doctor, I was hardly at home. Till my daughter Anjana (Anju) was about three years old, I would hardly get to see her, because I would leave home early and return home late, and both times she would be fast asleep. We work six days a week, so Saturdays, too, went in the same manner. On most Sundays, I would be busy lecturing, doing research or attending conferences which were invariably in other parts of India or abroad.

One day, Anju looked at me straight in my eye and asked, 'Who are you?' I was shocked and shaken to the core. That night I spoke my heart out to Rema, a completely shattered and disillusioned man. Calm as usual and without pointing a finger at me, she said, 'Mohan, this is what happens if you don't spend time with the family. To Anju, you are a stranger as you hardly spend any time with her.' I decided that it was time I make up to my daughter. Luckily, at this time, we could take a sabbatical abroad.

The next two years of our life, the first of which we spent at London and then Germany, I ensured I spent quality time with

Anju. I would get her ready for school, drop her off, pick her up, feed her and also read stories to her at night. These bedtime stories became a ritual, which would continue for many years. It was then that I realized the value of a work–life balance and how important it was to spend time with the family.

After Rema's untimely death in 2011, Anju and I decided that we would spend even more time with each other. She said to me, 'Papa, make a bucket list of the places you want to see and let's go see all of them one by one.' Thereafter, every year, we make it a point to take a holiday, usually in some exotic part of the world. This allowed me to spend time with Anju, my son-in-law, Ranjit, and my grandson, Pranav, whom I have got extremely attached to.

Whatever one may achieve in life, if it's without the support of one's family, it is simply not worth it. I have been blessed to have the support of my family, from the beginning of my career—starting with my father, Dr M. Viswanathan, who was my medical guru and mentor and who is mentioned several times in the book. My mother, Sarada, was a homemaker and the glue that held us all together. She brought up her five children with such love and affection that we blossomed as a family. I owe a lot of who I am today to the love and support of my mother.

All my siblings have been a great source of support to me. My elder sister, Shobana, is a diabetes educator and a psychologist, who went on to do her PhD. Her husband, Dr A. Ramachandran, is one of India's top diabetologists, and I had the opportunity to work with him for nearly twenty years in my early years spent at my father's centre. My younger brother, Arun, is the personification of love and a gentle and kind human being loved by everyone. My younger sister, Indira, migrated to the US, where she completed her PhD, and has done some outstanding research on diabetes. And finally, my youngest brother, Dr Vijay, is a very well-known diabetologist and now runs my father's hospital in Royapuram. Vijay is a close collaborator of mine in many diabetes-related projects. The spouses and children of my siblings have also been a great source of support to us at all times.

When Rema was first diagnosed with cancer, she requested her younger sister, Rekha, who was then living in the US, to return to India to help run our organization. Rekha immediately obliged, giving up her job with her husband to join us. Rekha slowly climbed the ladder and became an excellent administrator. After Rema's death, she served as the CEO of our organization and contributed greatly to the growth and development of the centre. Rekha, an extremely kind-hearted person, won the love and affection of all our staff, with whom she has maintained a very close rapport. It is the support provided by Rekha which helped us through the difficult times after Rema's death. One of Rema's brothers, Praveen, lives in Chennai and looks after all our printing needs so efficiently, while her other brother, Pradeep, lives in Canada. Both are pillars of strength to us.

I believe that whatever success we achieve in life is mostly due to the circumstances we are placed in and the support of our family and friends.

I have been blessed with the love and support of not only my immediate family but my 'extended family' as well—the staff at our various institutions. In the first two decades of my work, this included my clinical and research staff at the M.V. Hospital for Diabetes and the Diabetes Research Centre in Royapuram, who are too numerous to be named here. However, I must mention Dr C. Snehalatha, our head of biochemistry at that time, who was one of my close collaborators in my early research.

In the second half of my life, it was the staff of Dr Mohan's Diabetes Specialities Centre, the Madras Diabetes Research Foundation, our Education Academy and all our other institutions, who are all more like family to me. Without their loyalty and constant support, none of the achievements outlined in this book would have been possible. A huge thank-you to Team Dr Mohan's! As I always say to you, *the best is yet to come!*

My research collaborators in the UK, the US, Canada, Australia, Europe and Asia are far too many to name individually. They believed in me, supported me and remain lifelong friends. Some of them have been named in this book but to each one of them I would like to say, *I loved every minute of working with you.*

My life would have been meaningless without my wife, Rema, who was everything to me—friend, lover, wife, collaborator, partner and, most importantly, my soulmate and conscience keeper. A lot of my success is due to her silent support; she often sacrificed her own career for my sake. I can never thank you enough, Rema.

My daughter, Anju, son-in-law, Ranjit and grandson, Pranav, are my world—*thank you* is too small a world for all the sacrifices you have made for me. Thank you for tolerating me. Anju and Ranjit, I can't tell you how proud I am of both of you.

In writing this book, I have got help from many people. I would be failing in my duty if I did not thank my dear friend and classmate Dr Nandagopal (Nandu), a plastic surgeon who lives in Toronto. Nandu read my early draft and gave me sound advice and sometimes some much-needed constructive criticism as well. Thanks, Nandu!

Another dear friend, Dr Naresh Kumar, took on the arduous task of checking every quote in the book and tracing its source. Thank you, Naresh, for your love and support.

Mr Srinivasan Sadagopan, another friend and a writer himself, gave me several great suggestions after reading an early draft, and I wish to thank him.

Ms Apekshita Varshney, a professional writer and editor, patiently went through the manuscript, helping me edit several parts of it to make the book more interesting and cutting out a lot of 'flab'. Thanks, Apekshita.

Several of my friends, colleagues and staff have toiled hard to help me with this book. I can't thank all of them due to the space constraint, but I must thank my secretary, Ms Valli, and my former PhD student Dr Bhavadharini Balaji (now living in Toronto), for their extensive secretarial support.

My friends Hari Baskaran and Nanditha Krishna gave me valuable tips about publishing a book.

Ms Tarini Uppal, editor at Penguin Random House India, and the entire Penguin team have been a great source of support and, more importantly, believed that this book would become successful, and I wish to thank them all. I would also like to thank my good friend Mr Vijay Kelkar for introducing me to Tarini.

A Note on the Author

Dr V. Mohan's name is synonymous with diabetes and diabetology in India. Dr Mohan started working and doing research on diabetes along with his father, Prof. M. Viswanathan, considered the 'Father of Diabetology' in India, as a second-year medical student, when he was just eighteen. There has been no looking back since then, and for nearly five decades, Dr Mohan has been consistently contributing to diabetes healthcare, research, education and charity. After working for twenty years with his father along with his late wife, Dr Rema Mohan, Dr Mohan established the well-known Dr Mohan's Group of Diabetes Institutions. This includes Dr Mohan's Diabetes Specialities Centre (the hospital wing), the Madras Diabetes Research Foundation (the research wing) and Dr Mohan's Diabetes Education Academy (the education wing).

Dr Mohan established one of the largest chains of diabetes centres in the world, with over forty-eight branches spread across thirty-two cities and eight states of India and which have treated nearly 900,000 diabetes patients. A prolific writer and researcher right from his undergraduate-medical-student days, Dr Mohan has a prodigious number of publications to his name, with over 1300 articles, research papers and chapters in textbooks. He is one of the few medical doctors with an h-index of 135 and over 134,000 citations—considered a stupendous achievement even for a full-time academic researcher. He also contributes extensively to charity and effortlessly combines spirituality with science.

The Gene: An Intimate History
Siddhartha Mukherjee

Spanning the globe and several centuries, *The Gene* is the story of the quest to decipher the master-code that makes and defines humans, that governs our form and function.

The story of the gene begins in an obscure Augustinian abbey in Moravia in 1856 where a monk stumbles on the idea of a 'unit of heredity'. It intersects with Darwin's theory of evolution, and collides with the horrors of Nazi eugenics in the 1940s. The gene transforms post-war biology. It reorganizes our understanding of sexuality, temperament, choice and free will. This is a story driven by human ingenuity and obsessive minds—from Charles Darwin and Gregor Mendel to Francis Crick, James Watson and Rosalind Franklin, and the thousands of scientists still working to understand the code of codes.

This is an epic, moving history of a scientific idea coming to life, by the author of The Emperor of All Maladies. But woven through *The Gene*, like a red line, is also an intimate history—the story of Mukherjee's own family and its recurring pattern of mental illness, reminding us that genetics is vitally relevant to everyday lives. These concerns reverberate even more urgently today as we learn to "read" and "write" the human genome—unleashing the potential to change the fates and identities of our children.

Majestic in its scope and ambition, *The Gene* provides us with a definitive account of the epic history of the quest to decipher the master-code that makes and defines humans—and paints a fascinating vision of both humanity's past and future.

Being Mortal: Medicine and What Matters in the End
Atul Gawande

Doctors are trained to keep their patients alive as long as possible. But they are never taught how to prepare people to die. And yet for many patients, particularly the old and terminally ill, death is a question of when, not if. Should the medical profession rethink its approach to them? And in what way? With aging populations and hospital costs rising globally, these questions have become increasingly relevant.

In his new book, Atul Gawande argues that an acceptance of mortality must lie at the center of the way we treat the dying. Using his experiences (and
missteps) as a surgeon, comparing attitudes toward aging and death in the West and in India and drawing a powerful portrait of his father's final years-a doctor who chose how he should go-Gawande has produced a work that is not only an extraordinary account of loss but one whose ideas are truly important.

Questioning, profound and deeply moving, *Being Mortal* is a masterpiece.

Better: A Surgeon's Notes on Performance
Atul Gawande

Nowhere is the drive to do better more important than in medicine, where lives are on the line with every decision. Atul Gawande's gripping stories take us to battlefield surgical tents in Iraq, delivery rooms in Boston, a polio outbreak in India, and malpractice courtrooms in the US. He discusses the ethical dilemma of lethal injections, examines the influence of money on modern medicine, and recounts the contentious history of hand-washing. And as in all his writing, he gives us an inside look at his own life as a surgeon.

The Checklist Manifesto: How to Get Things Right
Atul Gawande

We live in a world of great and increasing complexity, where even the most expert professionals struggle to master the tasks they face. Longer training, ever more advanced technologies—neither seems to prevent grievous errors. But in a hopeful turn, acclaimed surgeon and writer Atul Gawande finds a remedy in the humblest and simplest of techniques: the checklist. First introduced decades ago by the U.S. Air Force, checklists have enabled pilots to fly aircraft of mind-boggling sophistication. Now innovative checklists are being adopted in hospitals around the world, helping doctors and nurses respond to everything from flu epidemics to avalanches. Even in the immensely complex world of surgery, a simple ninety-second variant has cut the rate of fatalities by more than a third.

In riveting stories, Gawande takes us from Austria, where an emergency checklist saved a drowning victim who had spent half an hour underwater, to Michigan, where a cleanliness checklist in intensive care units virtually eliminated a type of deadly hospital infection. He explains how checklists actually work to prompt striking and immediate improvements. And he follows the checklist revolution into fields well beyond medicine, from disaster response to investment banking, skyscraper construction, and businesses of all kinds. An intellectual adventure in which lives are lost and saved and one simple idea makes a tremendous difference.

Complications: Notes from the Life of a Young Surgeon
Atul Gawande

Atul Gawande performs surgery on medicine itself, laying bare a science that is complicated, perplexing and profoundly human. Dramatic true stories explore how mistakes occur, why good surgeons go bad, and what happens when medicine comes up against the inexplicable: an architect with incapacitating back pain but no physical cause; a young woman with nausea that won't go away; a TV newscaster whose blushing is so severe that she cannot do her job.